THALIA:
¡BELLEZA!

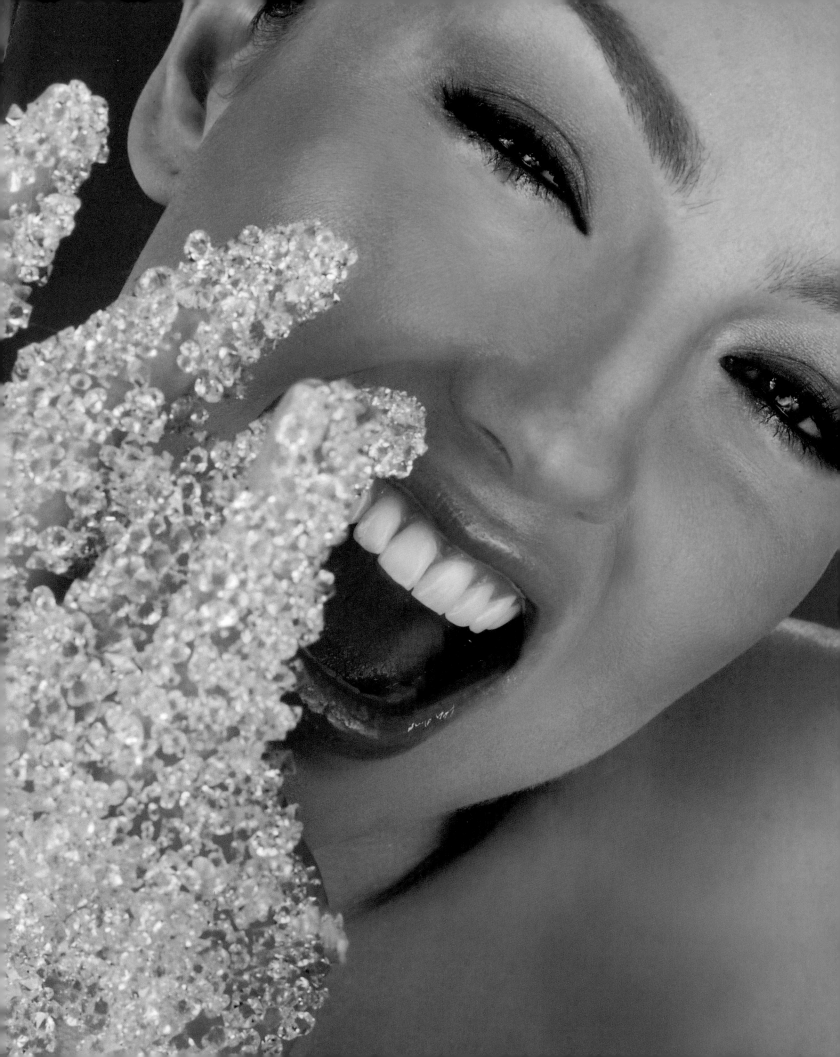

THALIA: ¡BELLEZA!

Lessons in Lipgloss and Happiness

BY THALIA

WITH BELÉN ARANDA-ALVARADO

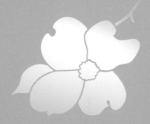

CHRONICLE BOOKS

SAN FRANCISCO

Page 207 constitutes a continuation of the copyright page.

Library of Congress Cataloging-in-Publication Data:

Thalía.
Thalia belleza! : lessons in lipgloss and happiness.
p. cm.
Includes index.
ISBN-13: 978-0-8118-5829-8
ISBN-10: 0-8118-5829-4
1. Beauty, Personal. 2. Cosmetics. 3. Beauty culture. I. Title.

RA778.T45 2007
646.7'2—dc22

2007016010

Manufactured in China
Designed by Sugar
Creative Director: Joanne Oriti

Distributed in Canada by Raincoast Books
9050 Shaughnessy Street
Vancouver, British Columbia V6P 6E5

10 9 8 7 6 5 4 3 2 1

Chronicle Books LLC
680 Second Street
San Francisco, California 94107
www.chroniclebooks.com

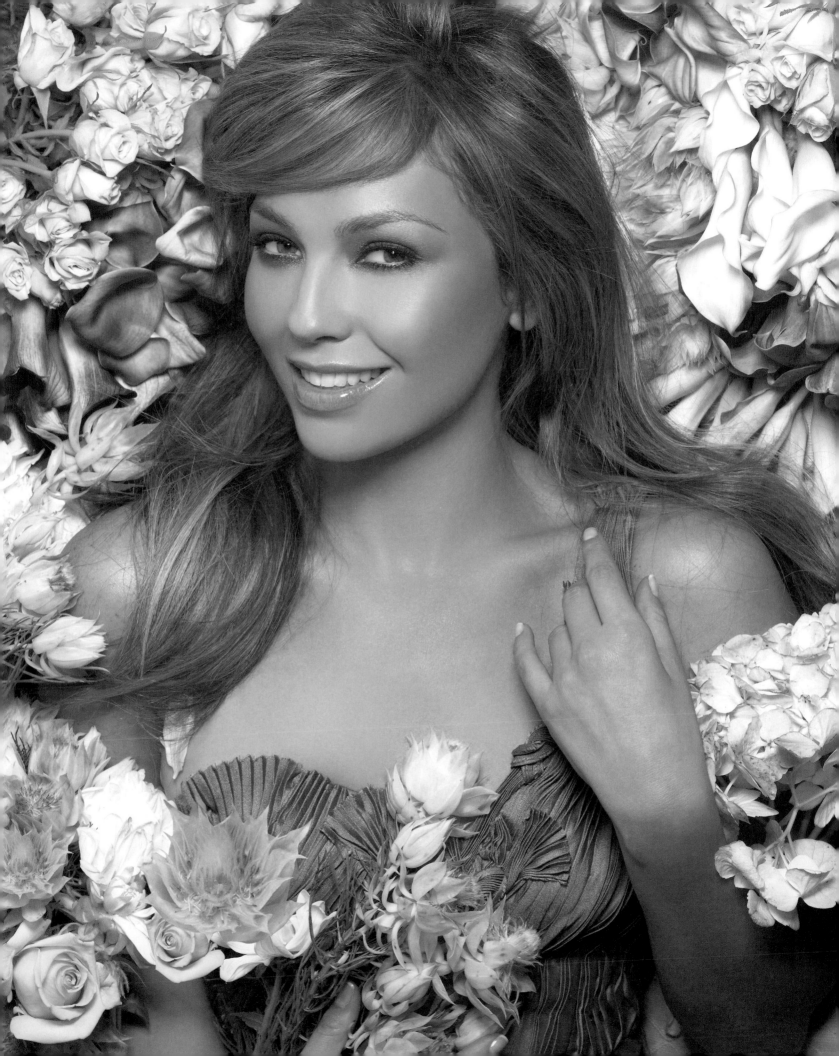

table of contents

My earliest beauty role model was my grandmother. Besides being hilarious, spry, and smart as a whip, she was the first person to teach me about taking care of myself, pampering my skin, and smelling wonderful. One of my first memories is of my abuelita running after me after I'd had my bath, a powder puff in hand, to tap sweet-smelling talc onto my pompis.

From my toddler years through my latest albums, videos, and fashion projects, you had better believe I've learned a thing or two about makeup, hair care, and fashion. But even more important to me are the lessons I've learned about feeling fabulous, becoming my "best self," and loving myself so much that I have the confidence to know what works for me and what doesn't.

My fans have watched me grow from a girl with braces, breakouts, and too much makeup to the jet-set chica I am today. I look better now, in my thirties, than I ever did before. This book is a guide to feeling your best. Express your beauty using all the tools at your disposal, be it a mascara wand or a fearless approach to life. ¡Viva la vida y vivela bella! ¡Orale!

Thalia

Foreword

Latin Beauty is a very specific type of beauty. I'm not suggesting that we're all one kind of beautiful. I know that, as Latinas, we come in different colors, shapes, and sizes. We come from different countries and we're very proud to be from that country. We have similar upbringings and similar cultures. Obviously, I'm proud to be a Latina. As different and individual as we all are, I think we definitely have a lot in common. When I think of Latina Beauty, I think of sexy, feminine, seductive, strong, nurturing women. We support, love, and flirt with our men like it's nobody's business! But, as much as we love being sexy and seductive with our men, there's nothing like the bond we share with our moms, sisters, and girlfriends—Latin girls like to stick by our girls. We love to talk openly about everything. We share our insecurities, our joys, our sorrows, and, most important, our beauty secrets.

When I think more about Latin Beauty, I (and many others) think of Thalia. I first met Thalia many years ago. She was on the phone with a mutual friend, when I asked "Who are you talking with?" the answer was "Thalia." No last name needed. Even though we'd never met I instantly said, "I love her, tell her I said Hi." Without skipping a beat, Thalia said "Daisy? Put her on!" So, here I was on the phone with one of the loveliest, sweetest, most genuinely fabulous girls I'd never met. It was as if we'd known each other for years, just a cool girlfriend. It wasn't until I got off the phone with her that I remembered she just happens to be a huge international superstar! As if that were not enough, she also comes from quite a pedigree of strong women…her mom, sisters—all powerhouses. So, who better to talk secrets with?

As a Latin woman myself, I know (OK, I was taught) the importance of feeling beautiful, and always being feminine. As just another girl, I know it's not as easy as it sounds. I, too, went through difficult stages, trying to figure out where I really fit in. I was born in Cuba, but I came to this country from Spain when I was 8. I didn't speak a word of English and because my Castellian accent (from Madrid) was so strong, the Latin kids in school didn't understand my Spanish either. Talk about culture shock. That's just the beginning, the rest of my life has been about figuring out who I really am. I'm a Latina, and although Spanish is my first language, I'm as "apple pie" as they come. It hasn't been easy finding my own look. Our society is so full of strong judgments, almost dictating what we should look like, eat, feel, even who we should be...needless to say it's easy to feel less than perfect. That's why I love what Thalia offers in this fantastic book. Not only does she show us how to get luscious lashes, cherubic cheeks, and plump pouts, she also gives us straight talk on how to work with what we've got. She's generous enough to share photos of some of her not-so-glamorous moments (yes, even she's had those) along with photos from the most important times of her life. She also makes over friends and family and shares her top tips from professional stylists. In this book she'll take you from basic makeup application to mind-body-spirit balance and back. She'll help you discover your own individual beauty.

Thalia is truly an inspiration to all of us who are on an endless quest for beauty inside and out.

— Daisy Fuentes

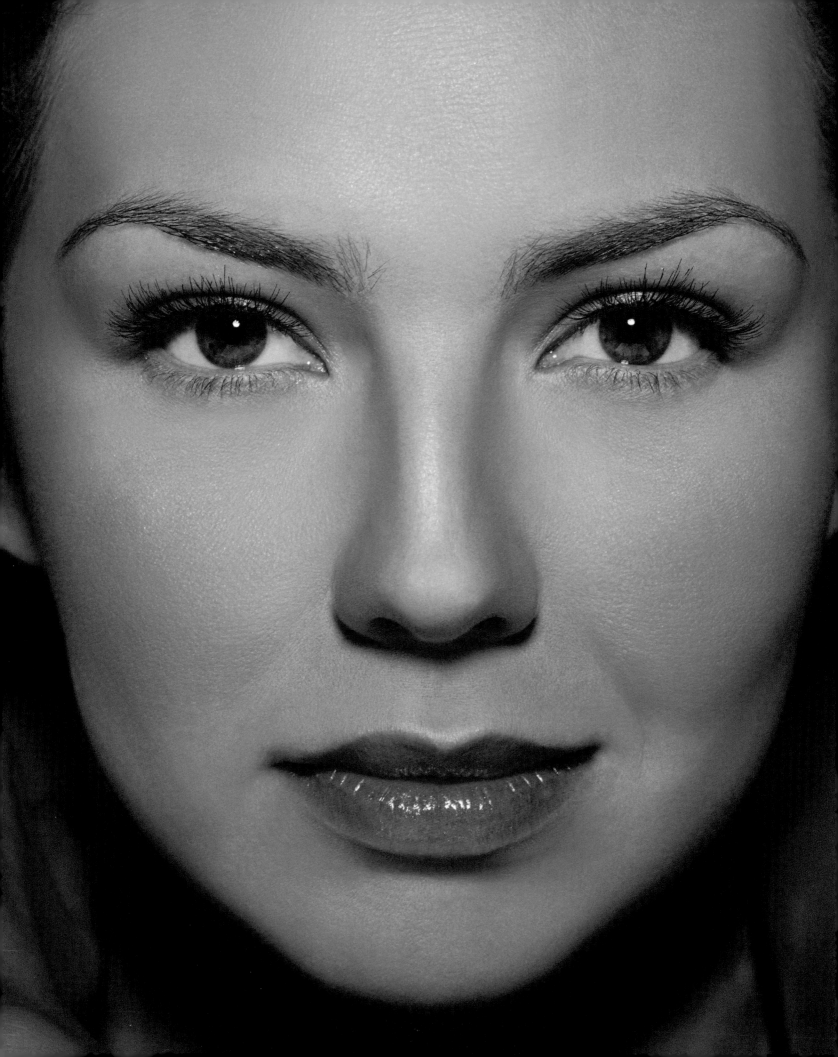

get glowing

SKIN CARE BASICS

When I was fifteen, two things happened in my life:

I became an official teen idol in Mexico with the premiere
of a telenovela entitled—appropriately—*Quinceañera*,
and I started what would be an ongoing battle with acne.
I developed blemishes that covered my forehead, my nose,
my chin, even my chest and my upper arms—and I have
the photos to prove it!

Of course, normal teen hormonal changes can provoke
the onslaught of acne, but I am convinced that my
battle with these blemishes erupted after a makeup
artist used brushes on me that had not been properly
cleaned. Ever since I made that connection, I've been
a fanatic about clean makeup brushes (I'm actually a
fanatic about cleanliness in general; I'm like the Mexican
Howard Hughes).

I tried everything to rid myself of acne, or at least cover
it up. I'd cut bangs in my hair that would fall strategically
over my blemished forehead—which only made things

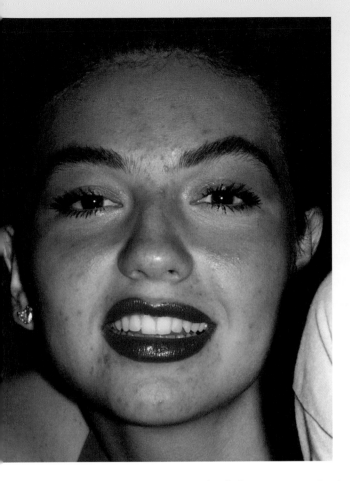

worse, since the natural oils from the hair-styling products exacerbated my acne. I bought every product I could get my hands on at the drugstore, and when they failed to help, I moved on to Accutane, an oral medicine that is available only by prescription. It's often the last resort for people with persistent acne like I had. It worked, but I still had to follow a strict skin-care routine.

In the end, I learned the hard way that there is only one effective weapon against bad skin: a beauty routine fine-tuned to your own personal skin type.

what is your skin type?

Skin types can vary throughout your life depending on your lifestyle and age. I've been almost every skin type there is. When I started to act in telenovelas, my skin became oily. The combination of the heavy makeup and hot studio lights was a recipe for disaster—it's like my skin was cooking under all that foundation, concealer, and powder! Later, after I tried all those treatments for acne, my skin became very dry. Now it has finally normalized, but I do suffer occasional bouts of sensitivity, especially around the nose, where I get some rosacea—an inherited gift from my mami. My multipersonality skin is a result of my crazy, busy life, but most women have one general skin type that changes slightly throughout the year, with the changes in seasons. The following list will help you determine your own skin type.

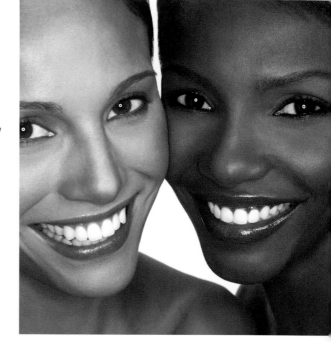

COMBINATION Dry cheeks and oily T-zone (forehead, nose, and chin), by far the most common skin type.

OILY Large pores and skin that appears to "absorb" makeup after only a few hours.

DRY Small pores and skin that feels tight after bathing and is prone to ashiness or blotchiness.

NORMAL Even skin tone with little blemishing or need for heavy moisturizers.

SENSITIVE Uneven skin tone and skin that tends to get easily irritated or inflamed and does not tolerate many skin-care products.

the right routine

It's best to tailor your skin-care routine to your skin type. The basics of any routine are to cleanse, tone, hydrate, and protect, which you should do at night and in the morning. Don't be afraid to change your routine if you see your skin is not responding the way it used to. Changes in seasons and climate can alter your skin-care needs dramatically. When I moved to New York from Mexico, I had to completely revamp my skin-care routine, because I had relocated from a climate that had two seasons to one that had four.

The skin type table on the following page outlines the types of products you should use in your skin-care routine, depending on your skin type.

skin type

SKIN CARE ROUTINE	COMBINATION	OILY	DRY	NORMAL	SENSITIVE
CLEANSE	gentle liquid cleanser	gel facial cleanser	cream cleanser	basic cleanser	fragrance-free cleanser
TONE	balancing toner	astringent to remove impurities	hydrating mist or lotion	non-alcohol-based toner	skip this step
HYDRATE	basic moisturizing lotion	water-based oil-free gel	cream formula	moisturizer in a lotion	fragrance-free lotion or cream
PROTECT	lightweight gel SPF of at least 15	oil-free or lightweight gel with SPF of at least 15	daily moisturizer with SPF of at least 15	daily moisturizer with SPF of at least 15	titanium or zinc oxide-based with SPF of at least 15

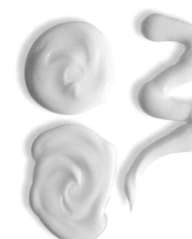

beauty boosters

The steps represented on the chart on page 15 are the bare minimum you need to do to keep your skin healthy. The following items are little details that make a big difference. If you incorporate them into your basic routine, you will go from healthy to glowing and radiant.

Eye cream should hydrate and pamper the delicate area around your eyes. I favor vitamin C–based formulas for their antioxidant (and therefore anti-aging!) properties.

Mattifying cream is a blessing for oily-skinned folks. It helps makeup hold and minimizes midday shine that comes from the oil glands on your nose, forehead, and chin.

Blotting papers are another boon for chicas with oily skin, because they absorb oil without rubbing away any makeup. They also help with makeup touch-ups. Some papers have a light coating of powder, so they absorb the excess oil from your skin while depositing powder to keep a fresh, even look.

Lightening lotion, applied in the morning and at night before you slather on your moisturizer, helps with manchas, the darker spots or areas on the face caused by sun damage, major hormonal changes (such as pregnancy), pimples, or bug bites. The only answer is regular spot application of a lightening lotion that lifts the darker pigmentation. The effects will be permanent on manchas left from bug bites or pimples. The darkened skin created by hormonal changes may reappear periodically. Avoid the sun during treatment, or the hormone- or sun-caused spots will reappear.

SKIN-CARE BUZZWORDS

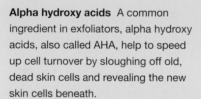

The language of skin care is more sophisticated than it used to be. Here are some key terms to know, since you might read these words on the bottles and boxes of new skin-care products.

Alpha hydroxy acids A common ingredient in exfoliators, alpha hydroxy acids, also called AHA, help to speed up cell turnover by sloughing off old, dead skin cells and revealing the new skin cells beneath.

Antioxidants The only known weapon against free radicals, antioxidants can mitigate the consequences of prolonged sun exposure. Common antioxidants include green tea, vitamin E, and vitamin C.

Beta hydroxy acid There is only one type of beta hydroxy acid: salicylic acid. It can penetrate oil, which means it can be effective for oily skin.

Collagen A protein present in the skin, collagen is responsible for the skin's elasticity and strength. As we age, our skin produces less collagen, which leads to the appearance of wrinkles.

Free radicals These suckers are our sworn enemy, because they accelerate the aging process. Sources of free radicals include cigarette smoke and UV light, but they are also produced naturally by our bodies, and they are present in pollutants that are common in the general environment. They work by damaging cell structures, which can in turn lead to precancers and cancers.

Glycerin An ingredient in many skin-care products, glycerin is a humectant, which means it attracts moisture from the environment.

Glycolic acid A form of AHA, glycolic acid is derived from sugarcane and grapes. It effectively penetrates the skin and, in high concentrations, is a key ingredient in doctor-administered chemical peels.

Hyaluronic acid This acid occurs naturally in our skin tissue, keeping it hydrated by attracting and retaining water. Skin-care products incorporate it because it "plumps" the skin.

Panthenol The ingredient listing for vitamin B_5, panthenol is commonly used in hair conditioners because it is the only vitamin that the hair can actually absorb. In skin-care products, panthenol is an effective emollient that soothes the skin.

Squalene Present in our own sebum— the oil our skin produces—squalene is also used in skin creams as a rich, nonirritating moisturizer.

sensitive skin rx

I went from acne-prone skin as an adolescente to sensitive skin as an adult, so my skin-care routine has been a figure-out-what-works-best process. But one thing that hasn't changed is my skin's sensitive side. An increasing number of women are finding that their skin has become more sensitive as well, either because of their overuse of exfoliating products or because of their environment. Things like the hole in the ozone layer that is getting larger every day don't help! Sensitive skin does need extra attention. Here are some tips that help me deal with mine:

Use only hypoallergenic and fragrance-free products on your face.

Use soothing, creamy cleaners that you can remove with a tissue rather than with water. When water evaporates from the skin, it leaves the skin feeling tight and even drier.

Apply hydrocortisone cream before bed for two to three days in a row, and you will notice less puffiness, a healing of red blemishes, and an improved evenness to the skin tone. Hydrocortisone helps to relieve inflamed skin, and it is available in over-the-counter creams that come in a tube. Personally, I like to apply something more natural, such as a cream with green tea, to help minimize inflammation.

Use an opaque concealer to cover red spots on the skin.

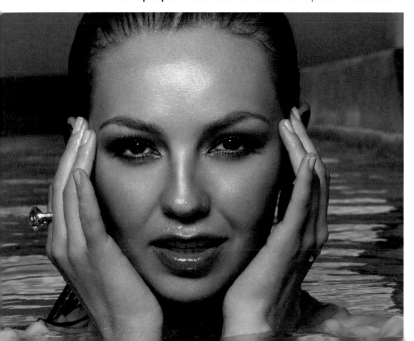

tips for hydrated, supple skin

I learned from all the talented facialists and aestheticians I have worked with that there is an art to skin care, from the way you clean your face to the way you take care of your lips.

Unless you have very oily skin, you may be able to skip cleansing in the morning. Instead, simply rinse the skin with water. If you find your face feels oily in the morning, keep washing. If your face feels tight, you can skip the soap-and-water routine. For me, when the weather is colder, I can get away with lightly wetting my skin with a washcloth dampened with warm water. On mornings when I wake up with oily skin, I know I have to wash with a cleanser and water.

If you have dry skin, you should use cream-based cleansers that can be removed with a tissue, rather than with water.

Use a mild, gentle exfoliator with very small particles to remove dry, dead skin cells. This will allow your moisturizer to penetrate evenly and effectively.

If you do wash with water, pat the skin with a towel afterward so it is damp, not dry. Then apply a generous amount of facial moisturizer to the still-damp skin. Concentrate on the cheeks and other areas where you feel tightness.

After you moisturize, wait five minutes before applying makeup, because moisturizer can leave the skin feeling tacky until it has been fully absorbed.

Look for moisturizers with hyaluronic acid, which plumps the skin by retaining water, or glycerin, which also keeps the skin's own moisture in.

Apply a richer moisturizer at night than you use during the day. In addition to hyaluronic acid and glycerin, other ingredients to keep an eye out for are squalene and panthenol.

During the winter months, use a humidifier at night to keep the air moist. I never owned one until I moved to New York, and now I take it with me everywhere. Sometimes I have two or three in a room. Humidifiers really work; I actually use them year-round, not just in the winter.

Eyes and lips are the most susceptible to changes in the weather and to dryness. I take extra care with these two areas of my face. Apply an eye cream in the morning and in the evening. Tap it on lightly with your ring finger to distribute it evenly and blend it in.

Exfoliate the lips with a gentle exfoliant. Follow with the thickest balm you can get your hands on. Look for one with botanical oils, petroleum jelly (yep, good ol' Vaseline), or shea butter. My personal always-works-without-fail option: Kiehl's Lip Balm.

Keep your hands away from your face! Your breakouts will abate if you stop touching your face. I promise!

CELEB SECRET REVEALED!

A movie-star beauty tip: A half teaspoon of sugar. A half teaspoon of olive oil. Mix well, and gently rub it on your lips. Remove with a tissue, and it will swipe away dead skin cells. Result? Lush, flawless, exfoliated labios worthy of a screen close-up.

removing makeup at night

I might have just returned from a twelve-hour flight that had been delayed six hours. The car may have been stuck in traffic for four hours on the way home. I might have a head cold, a headache, and sleep deprivation. The world could be coming to an end—and I would still take off my makeup and wash my face before I went to bed. To make it easy, I keep on hand the tools to help make the process quicker. I am loyal to Lancôme's Bi-Facil oil-based makeup remover for my eye makeup. Apply this with a cotton ball, and all your makeup, including your mascara, will slide off with minimal effort. To quickly clean my face, I use LaRoche-Posay's Demal Netoyant, which I can apply to my skin and quickly wipe off with a warm washcloth. Keeping some disposable moist towelettes handy also helps. That way, you won't even need water to wash your face anymore, so there is simply no excuse for skipping it. Make this a must-do, and soon you will start to enjoy taking care of yourself. Think of it as the last pampering step you take before you fall into a deep, well-deserved beauty sleep.

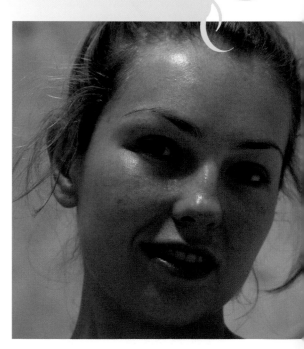

necessary pampering

Every señorita needs a little professional care once in a while. For the ultimate in skin care, treat yourself to a facial. I get a facial once a week, if I have the time. When I'm in nomad mode—that is, doing promotions or on tour—I get one at least once a month. When I was doing telenovelas, I had deep-cleansing facials twice a week because of all the heavy makeup and my acne. At the very least, a woman should treat herself to a deep-cleansing facial with the change of seasons, since a change in the weather and environment takes its toll on the skin. A good aesthetician will also give you advice on how to tweak your routine. If you have never had a facial, you might be overwhelmed by the many options available and the newfangled, ingredient-driven facials that promise to do all sorts of things. Here are the two main types you need to know about:

DEEP-CLEANSING FACIAL This usually involves a step in which the pores are opened or softened (usually with a combination of steam and massage), after which the facialist performs an extraction, which basically means taking out all of the gunk that is stuck in your pores. This is not particularly relaxing. For me, sometimes it was even painful. I developed a thick skin—pardon the pun—because I was doing it so often. If you have never had a deep-cleansing facial before, it can hurt, and it certainly can leave the skin feeling irritated. Extractions are typically done with a small metal tool called a comedone extractor. It looks like a little torture device. This is the type of facial that is often cryptically described in spa brochures as "bringing impurities to the surface." Translation: you may experience breakouts for a week or so afterward, so schedule your facial well in advance of any big event.

HYDRATING FACIAL This is a much more relaxing facial and my favorite in the winter months, or whenever my skin feels tired or looks dull. The steps in this facial are all geared toward pumping up the moisture level in your skin and usually involve a gentle exfoliation to reveal fresh, smooth skin, followed by a rich and creamy mask that feels delicious. The details and the steps may differ from spa to spa, but the end result should be the same. Think of it as giving your skin a big, fresh glass of water. Your face will look more radiant and rested afterward.

tips for young-looking skin

Don't drink, don't smoke, and don't tan. ¡Que aburrida! But you know what? Abstaining works. Booze, cigarettes, and too much sun all will make you look old very quickly. They let aging free radicals run amok in the cells of your skin. The skin is the largest organ of your body. Take care of it.

Moisturize, moisturize, moisturize! The goal here is to keep the skin hydrated and soft, not to slather on greasy creams that will not let the skin breathe.

Use sunblock religiously. I use a separate sunblock for my SPF protection. Although many foundations now incorporate SPF into the formula, I prefer to use a separate sunblock, which I can reapply as needed. The SPF needs to be 30 or higher—I personally never leave the house without a 60—and it needs to protect you from the sun's UVA (aging) and UVB (burning) rays. These are commonly described as "broad spectrum" or "full spectrum" sunblocks. If you don't like the idea of putting so many things on your face, try to use a moisturizer that has an SPF, instead of piling on moisturizer, sunblock, and a separate foundation. My sunblock of choice is Anthelios by La Roche–Posay. In the States you can get it in an SPF 15, but I use the higher formulas (at least 60) that I can purchase in Latin America and Europe.

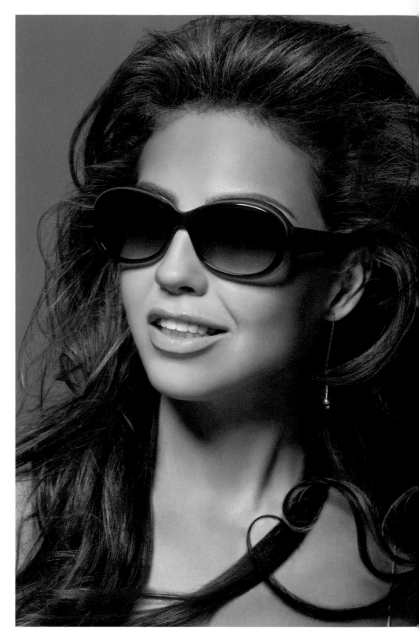

Keep a pair of dark sunglasses nearby at all times. In addition to using sunblock daily, wearing sunglasses helps prevent the crow's-feet wrinkles you get from squinting in the sun. Wearing sunglasses is an easy way to look instantly chic, as well as nonchalant in the face of paparazzi who jump out of nowhere to take your picture.

I believe in antioxidants, and I look for creams for my face and for my eyes that have antioxidants such as vitamin C, vitamin E, or green tea.

Use illuminating or light-diffusing foundation for your skin. These brighten the skin and minimize the appearance of fine lines—I will get into more detail about this in the next chapter.

glow on the go

With all the touring I do, it seems I've spent a good chunk of my life in airplanes. Because the air on planes is dry and recycled, it can wreak havoc on a girl's complexion. I do everything I can to protect my skin in the air. In addition to my cashmere blanket, a pair of slippers, a mini lint roller (to pick up the residual hairs or dead skin cells of the previous passenger—that's my neatnik side), I also carry on with me these items:

A facial mister filled with pure spring water.

Water to drink for every hour I spend in the air.

A creamy moisturizer to keep my skin hydrated and protect it from environmental stressors in the icky recirculated airplane air.

Two vitamin C tablets and some echinacea, to boost my immune system.

Antibacterial hand wipes. And I keep my hands away from my face.

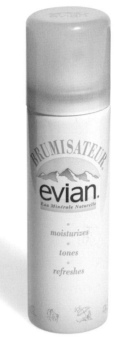

MY MAMI TOLD ME ...

Never pick at your blemishes.

Never go to bed with makeup on.

Never ignore your neck: the routine for the face should extend to the neck.

Never leave the house without sunblock on your face, neck, chest, and hands.

...and she was right!

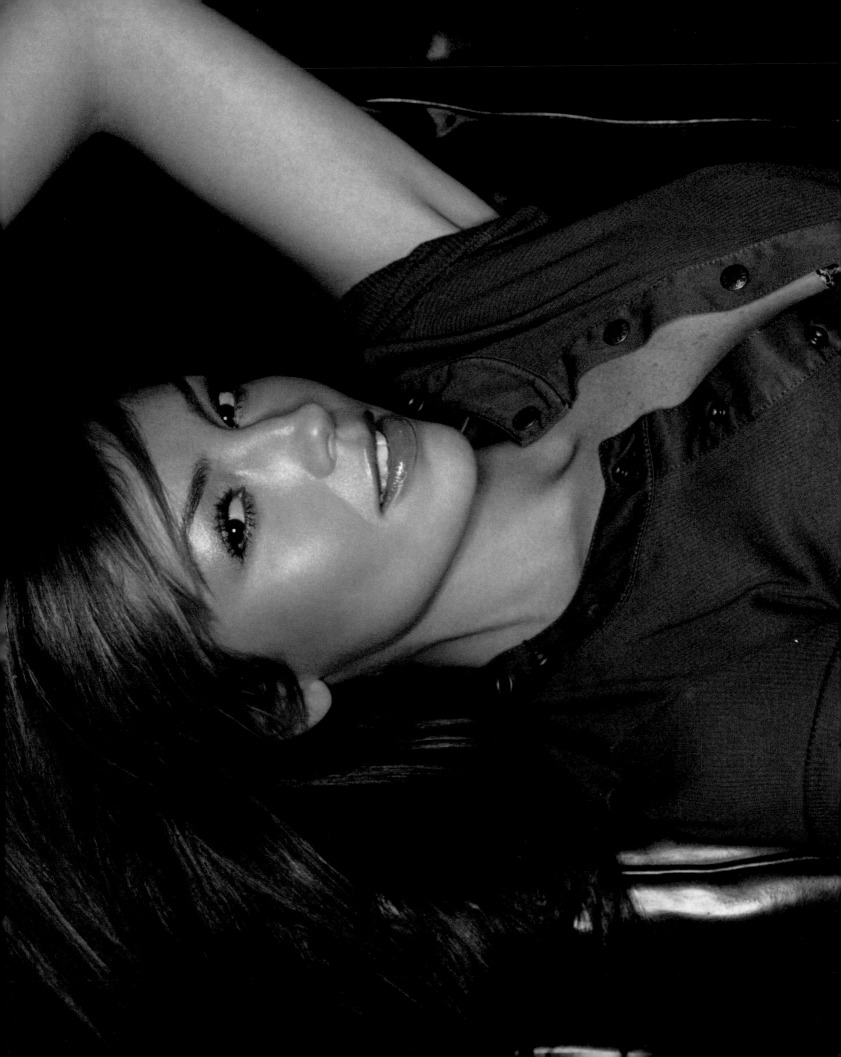

laying a great foundation

BASE, CONCEALER, AND POWDER

When I first started working on telenovelas and singing on stage, the trend in makeup application was heavy foundation. At the time, everyone from Cindy Crawford to Cyndi Lauper was sporting that super-matte, very opaque, heavy-handed masklike look. I made the same mistake. My makeup artist gave me three Angel Face pancake shades to choose from—pink, pinker, and pinkest. The result: my face looked one color, and my body looked another. Finding my true color—a frustration most women can relate to—took time and practice. I had to learn how to use concealer and foundation to make my skin look healthy, luminous, and vibrant.

Today, women of all shades have the opposite problem. The beauty industry has recognized the diversity of skin tones and the beauty needs of all of us. (This is good.) The end result: tons of options and myriad choices. (This is confusing.) I'll help you cut through the clutter. But first, a word on tools.

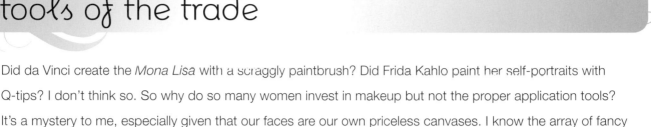

tools of the trade

Did da Vinci create the *Mona Lisa* with a scraggly paintbrush? Did Frida Kahlo paint her self-portraits with Q-tips? I don't think so. So why do so many women invest in makeup but not the proper application tools? It's a mystery to me, especially given that our faces are our own priceless canvases. I know the array of fancy tools of the trade can feel intimidating and overwhelming, but it's really quite simple to stock your makeup bag. Here are my essentials:

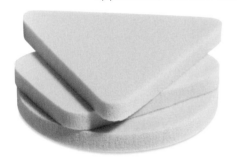

FOUNDATION SPONGES There are various shapes and sizes of foundation sponges. I prefer the angled sponges over the round, since the angles of the sponges make it easy to get into creases around the mouth and nose. These sponges are also multifunctional: I use them to blend base, shading, and bronzer, for spot application, and also when applying body makeup to my legs or décolletage. When I am using the foundation sponge to apply my base, I wet the sponge with water and squeeze it out until the sponge remains damp and soft. Applying makeup with a damp sponge makes blending easier. Powder foundations usually come in a compact with a sponge that you can use wet or dry. If you apply powder foundation with a damp sponge, the coverage is not as heavy. If you apply it with a dry sponge, then the coverage is heavier. You can wash and reuse sponges, but discard them once they start to disintegrate.

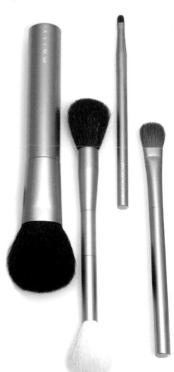

MAKEUP BRUSHES When I buy makeup brushes, I look for natural bristles and a compact shape. Avoid brushes with stray or uneven bristles. You'll find countless styles and a wide variety of price points for makeup brushes on the market—from the ultra-expensive Kevyn Aucoin sable-hair brushes to miniature, easy-to-carry brush kits from Sephora—that you can tuck away in your purse. Here are the ones I keep in my makeup bag to look my best. From left to right:

❋ Loose powder brush: big and fluffy for all-over application.

❋ Highlight/contour/blush brush for the cheeks: the light bristles are for the highlighter, the dark bristles for the contour and blush.

❋ Small eye-shadow brush: for applying contour shadow or to create smoky eyes with your eye shadow.

❋ Large eye-shadow brush: for applying all-over color to the ball and the upper lid.

❋ Lip brush (not shown): stiff and pointed for precision.

EYELASH CURLER Feel intimidated or have visions of pulling out your eyelashes by accident? Get over it, and get yourself an eyelash curler. It's truly a woman's best friend. I simply can't understand why everyone does not have one. You can now purchase anything, from an extra-fancy, heated, gold-toned eyelash curler that promises to give you nonstop eyelash curling all the way down to a very basic, take-with-you mini eyelash curler that folds up easily into your makeup bag and are available at most drugstores. The point—there is no excuse not to have one and use it! Keep it clean and bacteria-free by cleaning or replacing the sponge that goes in the curler. With a few seconds' use of an eyelash curler, your lashes go from barely there to fabulously flirty. Your eyes will look bigger, brighter, and more alluring.

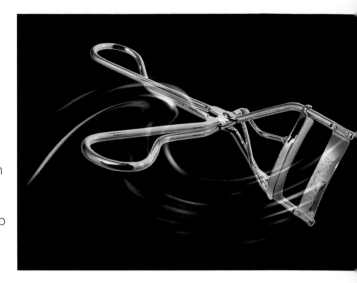

caring for your makeup brushes

Call me a demanding diva or a cabrona—I don't care—but I will not compromise when it comes to clean makeup brushes. Makeup brushes are like petri dishes—breeding grounds for bacteria, viruses, and all sorts of icky things. At a photo shoot, I expect the makeup artist to show me that he or she has a new, unused set of brushes on hand before he or she so much as puts a single stroke of makeup on my face. As I mentioned earlier, I am convinced that my ongoing battle with acne was caused in part by dirty makeup tools.

For regular cleansing of my makeup brushes, I use Johnson's baby shampoo. For more rigorous cleaning, I use Shu Uemura's brush cleanser. Both of these are strong enough to kill any germs or bacteria but gentle enough to keep the natural hair bristles from drying out. They also work well if you have sensitive skin and are worried that dyes, detergents, or heavy fragrances will irritate your skin. Cleansing your makeup brushes removes built-up excess makeup and oils that the bristles pick up from your skin. You should clean your brushes every three or four months. (I wash mine every month!) Here's how:

Dampen the bristles under running water.

Apply a drop of cleanser into the palm of your hand, then gently swipe the brushes back and forth over your palm. The bristles should become sudsy, but don't rub them too vigorously.

Holding the brushes upside down, rinse the bristles in running water until the water runs clear.

After cleaning and rinsing, fill your wash basin with warm water and add a drop of hair conditioner to the water. Dip the brushes in the water for a few seconds, then empty the basin and rinse the brushes.

Once the brushes are clean, gently squeeze out any excess water.

Place the brushes on a paper towel and allow them to dry completely (I leave them overnight) before using them again.

When not in use, store brushes in a makeup case, so that the bristles remain flat. This helps to ensure that the brushes maintain their overall shape.

packing your pretties

This is a motto I live by: A place for everything and everything in its place. This applies to everything I own, including my beauty goodies. I have a great system for organizing my makeup, which makes it easy for me when I am on tour, doing promotions, or anytime I'm in a hurry: I have a different-color makeup bag for each area of my face. For example, I have a purple eye makeup bag, which holds my eyelash curler, my tweezers, my brow powder and pencils, all my eye brushes, and all of my eye makeup. I keep a red bag for my lips, with balm, lip brush, lip-pencil sharpener, and every lip color you can imagine, and a green bag for my cheeks. This way, I know on sight what to reach for, so I am not fumbling around for my lip color before I rush out the door.

foundation fundamentals

I have had the Victoria's Secret preferred makeup artists work wonders on my face. Angelina Jolie's top beauty team has glammed me up. I have had my makeup done by Beyoncé's lethal weapon of a makeup artist. My hair has been straightened, curled, and styled at the hands of J.Lo's favorite hairdresser Oribe. The fabulous Troy Surratt—the right-hand man of the legendary makeup artist Kevyn Aucoin—has primped and prettied me up for many photo shoots. Working with all of these top people allowed me to learn the best practices of beauty, which I bring to you here in this book. What was one thing they all swore by? The fact that foundation and concealers are the must-know beauty fundamentals for a great face.

Foundation should be used to even out general discoloration in the skin tone. It is best to begin with base before proceeding to blush or contouring or other makeup, because foundation creates the "smooth canvas" that the rest of your makeup is applied to. You can expect a good foundation to minimize discoloration in the skin and mute the appearance of pimples and dark spots, but it won't cover them completely; that is what a concealer is used for.

At the same time, foundation is not a must-use for all women. If you have even-toned

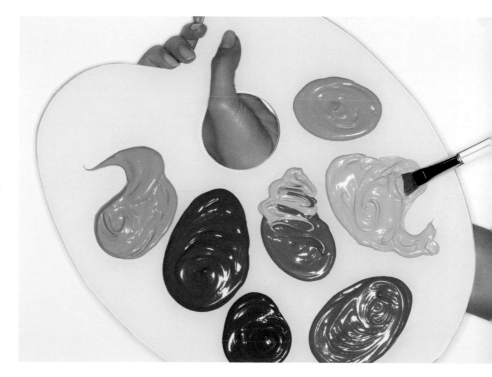

skin, you can actually skip this step and instead rely on concealer to cover up certain areas (typically the undereyes and the reddish or darker areas around the nose and chin). This is what I do for everyday wear—I use a concealer to cover up my little flaws, then I go on with the rest of my makeup.

Foundations now promise to do all sort of things, from absorbing oil to making your skin look younger to preventing pimples. Many foundations now also come with sunscreen in the formula. This is a great add-on, but as I explained in the section on moisturizers, I like to use an additional, separate sunblock with a strong SPF. This is because even if you don't wear foundation—because you can get away with only concealer or you just opt to go makeup-free—you still need to protect your skin from the sun. Also, unlike foundation, you may want to reapply sunblock throughout the day. It's easier to do that with just a sunblock, instead of reapplying foundation.

selecting the right foundation

If you take only one thing away from this chapter, let it be this: your foundation should match the color that your skin *is*, not the color that you want your skin to be. That's the most important aspect of foundation. Even if you can choose the right formula and apply it flawlessly, unless you have the right shade, your foundation and any makeup you apply afterward will look awful. I hate it when I see beautiful niñitas with "chin straps"—those awful demarcating lines under the chin that show where the foundation ends and where the real skin begins. It makes me want to run up to them with a foundation sponge in hand, yelling, "Blend, carajo, blend!"

Because choosing the right shade is so critical, I recommend you go to a beauty counter in a well-lit store for help. A competent cosmetics specialist will ask the right questions to help you determine which formula will work best. She will ask about your skin type and how much coverage you want, and she'll direct you to the line that best suits your needs. Then the two of you can work together to find the best color. When looking at the color options from a foundation line, choose the shade you think will work best on your skin, then select one shade lighter and one shade darker. Apply the three shades to your lower cheek, near the jawline. The shade that most closely matches your skin tone wins.

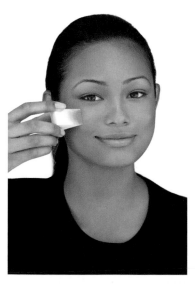
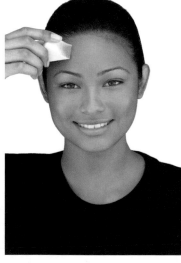

applying your foundation

Foundation should enhance your skin tone, not change it or cover your skin like a mask. With the right foundation and the right application techniques, no one will know that you're wearing it. That's the goal.

Clean, moisturize, and apply sunblock to your face. No foundation looks good on dry skin. Allow the moisturizer and sunblock to be fully absorbed before you begin applying the foundation.

Wet your foundation sponge with water, and squeeze out any excess: the sponge should be damp, not dripping.

Apply the foundation on the palm of your hand, then dab the sponge over the foundation, allowing the foundation to penetrate the sponge.

Apply the foundation to your skin with the sponge, using a quick dab and roll motion, starting with your cheek, your forehead, and your chin. Apply it evenly, and blend, carajo, blend! Be especially careful along the hairline and jawline and in the crevices around the mouth and nose. Use the narrow sides of the foundation sponge for smoothing over your whole face, and the edge tips for the crevices. The final look should be a smooth, even canvas on the skin.

Blend the foundation far down enough along the jawline to ensure a seamless transition between your face and the front of your neck. This is why it's critical to get foundation that matches your actual skin tone: otherwise it will look weird wherever the foundation ends and your real skin begins.

foundation chart

Foundations come in three types of coverage or opacity levels. Minimal coverage will give a gentle evening-out effect to the skin tone. Medium coverage is better for skin with larger blotchy patches such as the nose, chin, or cheeks. High coverage is a must for mujeres with lots of discoloration, inflammation, or uneven pigment.

TINTED MOISTURIZER	LIQUID	MOUSSE	POWDER	CREAM OR STICK
coverage: minimal	*coverage:* medium	*coverage:* medium	*coverage:* medium if applied with a damp sponge; high when applied with a dry sponge	*coverage:* high
best for: normal skin with even skin tone	*best for:* normal to oily skin	*best for:* normal to dry skin	*best for:* very oily skin, blotchy skin	*best for:* dry skin with discoloration

In a rush? After you have applied your foundation, place a tissue lightly over your face to absorb any excess foundation or moisture. Then move on to the rest of your makeup application.

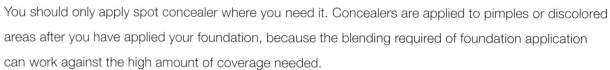

concealers

You should only apply spot concealer where you need it. Concealers are applied to pimples or discolored areas after you have applied your foundation, because the blending required of foundation application can work against the high amount of coverage needed.

concealer chart

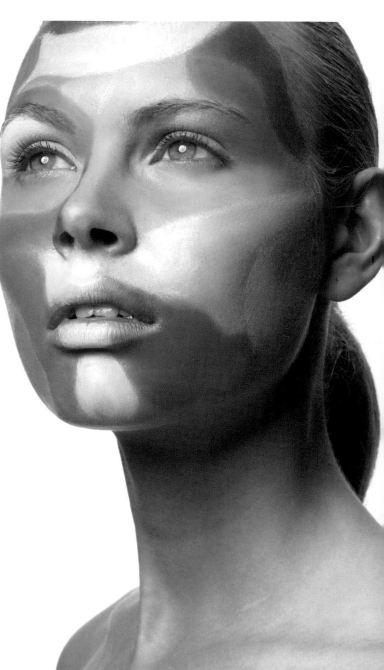

LIQUID	ILLUMINATING CONCEALER
coverage:	*coverage:*
minimal	medium
best for:	*best for:*
under the eyes; apply it over eye cream	under eyes (I swear by Touché Éclat by Yves Saint Laurent. ¡Me encanta!)
STICK	**CREAM**
coverage:	*coverage:*
high	high
best for:	*best for:*
very dark eye circles, areas of redness	blemishes

TOOLS To use a concealer to best advantage, you'll need these tools:

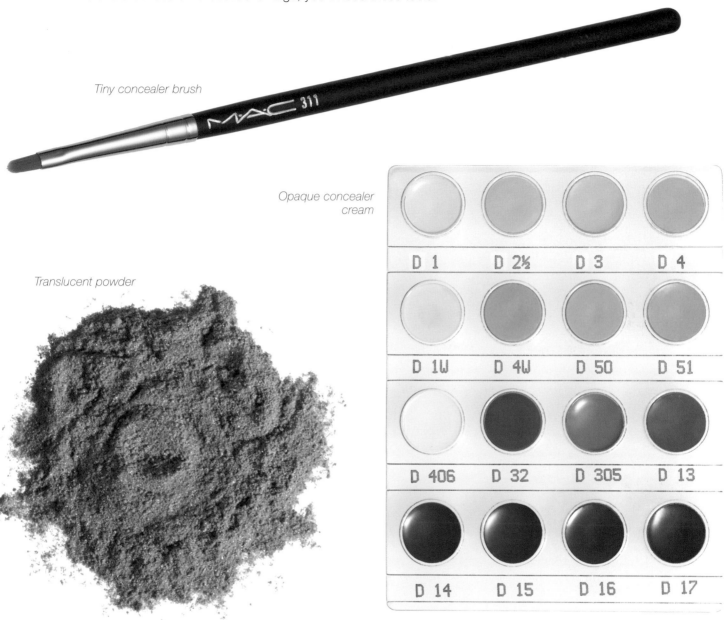

Tiny concealer brush

Opaque concealer cream

Translucent powder

D 1	D 2½	D 3	D 4
D 1W	D 4W	D 50	D 51
D 406	D 32	D 305	D 13
D 14	D 15	D 16	D 17

TECHNIQUE For a concealer to work its magic, start with one that is a shade lighter than your own skin tone or a shade that matches your skin tone exactly. I like a concealer palette like the one shown above, so I can mix and blend the colors to get the exact shade I need. Use your hand as your painter's palette: dab the different shades onto your hand and blend until you get the right color.

"Pointilism" is how I describe a blemish concealer technique that a makeup artist taught me. And thank God for that! I don't care if you are in your teens or in your forties—breakouts suck! As a former acne sufferer, I have found this technique to be a real face-saver, because breakouts stop for no one and nothing—not for big awards shows, or big wedding days, and especially not the pesky paparazzi. Pointilism helps give me an airbrushed, Photoshopped, flawless look—and I still look like me!

❋ Using the small end of a concealer brush, apply a small amount of concealer cream on top of and around the pimple or blemish.

❋ Use the brush to blend the concealer well.

❋ For larger pimples, use the other tip of the concealer brush—literally, the end of the brush handle—to "spackle" concealer around the pimple. You are blending the edge of the concealer without touching the top of the pimple. This helps to minimize, ever so slightly, the raised look of a pimple. Use the end of the brush handle to gently apply and spread the concealer.

❋ When a pimple is muy rebelde, or very stubborn and yucky, try the above technique, and follow with a thin coat of translucent powder applied using the small pointed concealer brush. Then, apply a second round of "spackle" concealer. This powder step will set, or "fix," the concealer over the pimple for long-lasting coverage.

❋ Apply a thin coat of translucent loose powder with a fluffy powder brush to set the concealer.

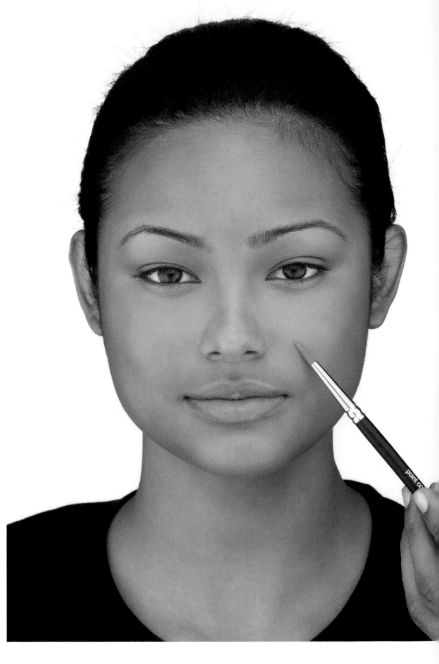

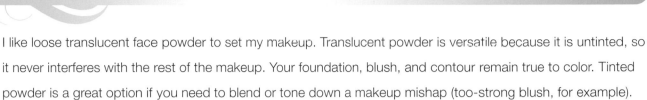

powder primer

I like loose translucent face powder to set my makeup. Translucent powder is versatile because it is untinted, so it never interferes with the rest of the makeup. Your foundation, blush, and contour remain true to color. Tinted powder is a great option if you need to blend or tone down a makeup mishap (too-strong blush, for example).

Apply either powder with a big, fluffy brush and you will create a smooth, flawless finish to your face: your skin will be ready for the magic of blush, bronzer, or whatever enhancement you choose. I use only pressed powder for a night out, and I keep a compact in my purse for touch-ups. The powder keeps my makeup in place and minimizes shine.

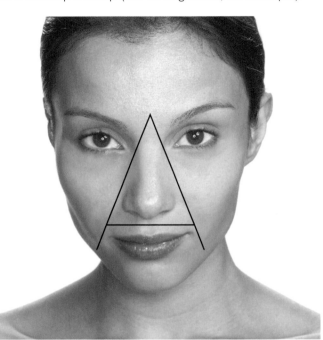

Apply powder in an A-shape as illustrated here to eliminate bad shine while still allowing your skin to remain fresh and dewy.

As important a tool as powder is, it can be equally important to know when *not* to use it. Only geishas and goths can rock the white doughboy look. Moments to avoid powder overload:

When you are trying to create a "dewy" look.

Over highlighter, since it will matte out the shine.

Before applying contour, because it is hard to blend after you have applied face powder.

Before applying cream blush, for the same reason as above.

If you have extremely dry skin, because powder will make your skin feel drier.

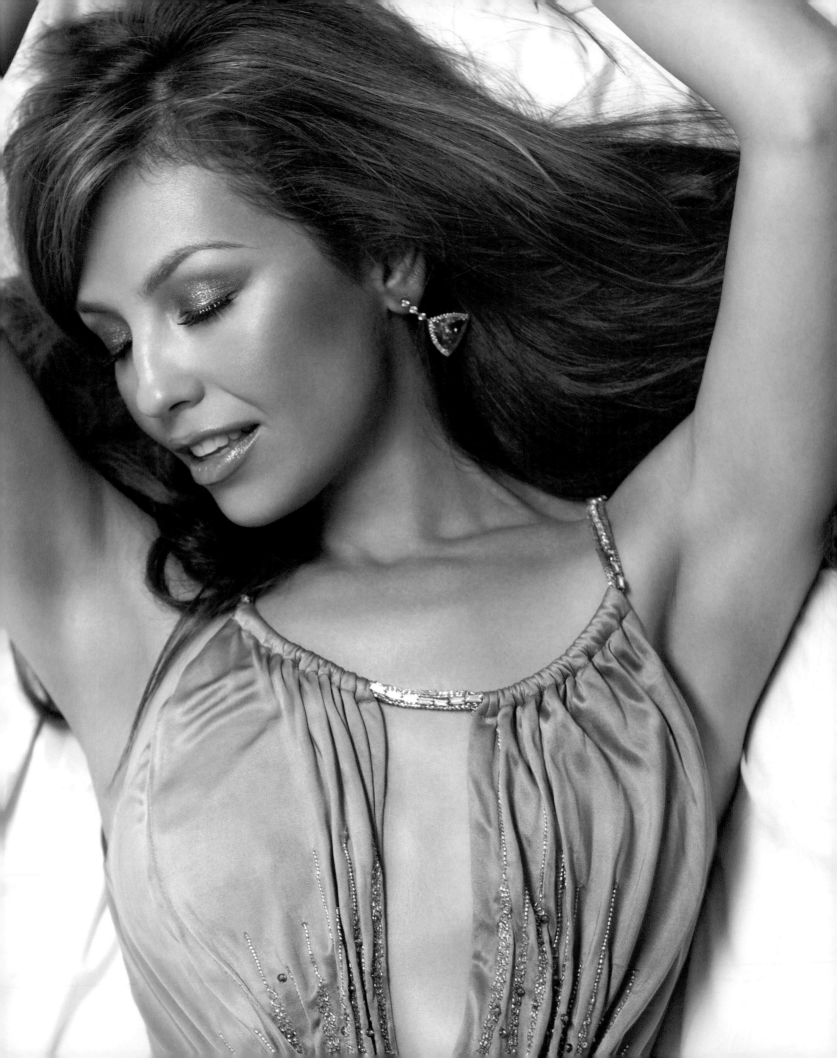

shape, color, and glow
SHADING, HIGHLIGHTER, BLUSH, AND BRONZER

What's the best proof that a new makeup technique is working? When people start speculating that you've had un arregladito—the euphemism for plastic surgery. That's what happened to me when I discovered how to shape and define my face. It was a revelation: All of a sudden I had cheekbones! The celebrity magazines had a field day. I read all about "reliable anonymous sources" who swore I'd gotten cheek implants, had a nose job, and bought a whole new set of teeth. I almost felt bad admitting that I'd actually achieved my new look with simple contouring, some highlighter, and a great blush.

My cheekbones were long hidden behind baby fat, or carita de niña. It wasn't until I reached my thirties that my cheekbones emerged. But trust me, my face still gets puffy when I eat too much Chinese takeout or I'm tired, so I have developed a couple of quick shaping techniques that work like a charm. Try them out and I swear people will ask if you've "had some work done"!

find your face

The trick of shaping and defining the face is to use color and makeup for an effect that is smooth and subtle. But first you need to understand what type of shape your face has. There is a saying that goes, "Sin mascaras, tiene que ser sincero antes del espejo," which means, "Without a mask, you must be honest in front of the mirror." In this spirit of beauty self-revelation and fearlessness, I'll be the first to admit that like many Latinas, I have a face that is as round as a pie. The good news is, this shape tends to lend a more youthful look. The bad news is, your cheekbones can be hard to find.

The shape of your face will affect your makeup technique and even your choice of hairstyle, so determining the shape is essential. Here is a quick chart to help you identify yours.

ROUND
(This is me!)

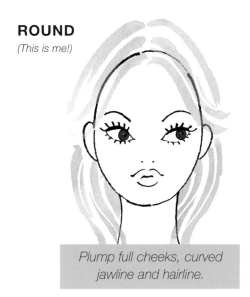

Plump full cheeks, curved jawline and hairline.

SQUARE

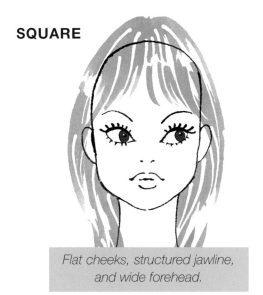

Flat cheeks, structured jawline, and wide forehead.

LONG

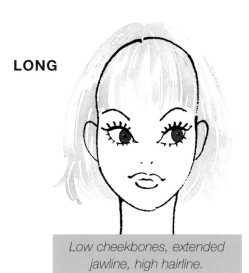

Low cheekbones, extended jawline, high hairline.

HEART

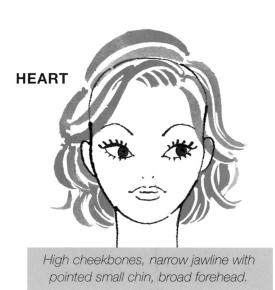

High cheekbones, narrow jawline with pointed small chin, broad forehead.

shaping products

Choices, choices, choices! So many different products have come on the market in the past few years, it's hard to know which ones to use. Highlighters and contours define the shape of your face. Bronzers and blush add color and sometimes a slight glow. Here are some important distinctions:

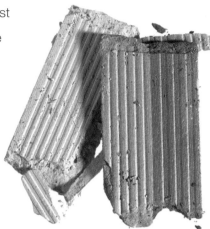

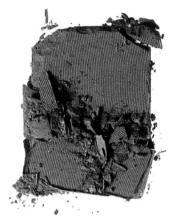

HIGHLIGHTERS These have luminescent particles that impart a slight sheen to the skin, but they do not necessarily add color to the face. Apply a highlighter to the part of your face you want to emphasize. I will show you when and how a little later.

CONTOURS These products should not be confused with bronzers or blush. Contour products are usually matte. You use them to shape your face. Apply contour on areas you want to deemphasize.

BRONZERS Sometimes these have shimmer in the formula. They are used to give a flash of color to the entire face. *Don't* use bronzers to shape your face, unless the glitter particles are small. The point of a contouring or shading product is to have the area where it is applied visually recede or seem smaller. The glitter particles in bronzers, which catch the light and draw the eye, have the opposite effect. Use these pearlescent bronzers the wrong way and you will look like a glowing balloon. These shimmery formulas are harder to use if you don't have a lot of experience. Matte bronzers are safer and can be used with highlighter, and you will still get a nice warm glow to the face. Apply a bronzer where the sun naturally hits your face: on your nose, cheekbones, chin, and forehead.

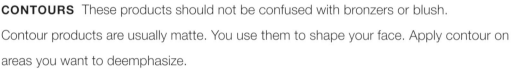

BLUSH These products come in many formulas (powder, gel, cream) and finishes (sheer, shimmery, matte), but they are always used for the same purpose: to give a flush of color to the cheeks, and only the cheeks. I usually use a bronzer and blush together, though many women opt out on the blush if they feel a bronzer is enough to give some color to the face. Blush should not be used to shape or define your features, which is what went wrong with the '80s makeup looks: women tried to use pink blush to carve out cheekbones. They just ended up looking like they had pink war paint on.

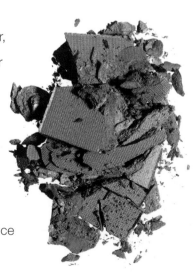

The following chart clarifies the different kinds of makeup you can use to define or enhance the shape of your face.

PRODUCT	TYPE	WHERE TO APPLY	HOW TO APPLY
HIGHLIGHTER	Liquid	Balls of the eyelids, brow bone, down the center of the nose, and a dot in the middle of the chin	Spot application with fingertips
	Cream	Same as above, and on larger areas such as the clavicle bone, the shoulders, cheekbones, on the bow of the lip, and on lips over lip color	With fingertips or a sponge
	Powder	On larger areas such as cheeks, the meaty area of the décolletage, shoulders, legs, and arms	With medium-size angled brush
CONTOUR	Cream	Hollows of the cheeks, jawline, hairline, sides of the nose, under chin, the center of the décolletage, under and over the clavicle bone	With damp sponge or foundation brush
	Powder	All areas you want to deemphasize. Powder is best for daily wear.	With medium- to small-size angled brush

(continued)

PRODUCT	TYPE	WHERE TO APPLY	HOW TO APPLY
BRONZER	Powder	Cheeks, forehead, chin (wherever the sun hits naturally), and a light dusting over the face, including neck and chest to add warmth	With blush brush
	Gel or stick	Cheeks, forehead, chin—wherever the sun hits	With fingertips
	Liquid	Cheeks, forehead, chin—wherever the sun hits	With fingertips; this is the hardest to blend
BLUSH	Powder	On the apples of the cheeks and across the bridge of the nose	With blush brush
	Cream	On the apples of the cheeks and across the bridge of the nose	With fingertips
	Gel	On the apples of the cheeks and across the bridge of the nose	With fingertips

shape shifting: working with the shape of your carita

Now that we have the different shapes and products explained, here is a quick reference list for which shaping techniques work best on which face shapes.

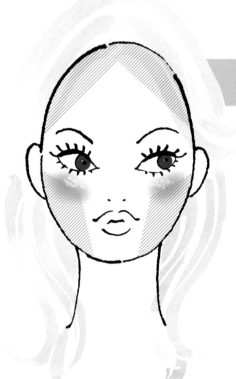

ROUND FACE *Your aim is to reduce the overall broadness of the face.*

Contour *Use in the hollows of the cheeks and along sides of forehead.*

Highlighter *Use above the apples of the cheeks and on the middle of the chin.*

Blush *Use along the cheekbone.*

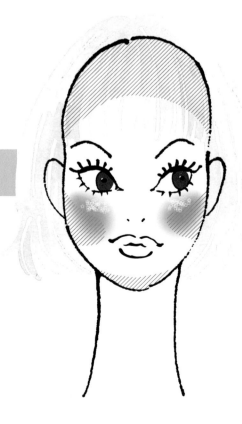

LONG FACE *The goal is to minimize the length of the face while maximizing the width.*

Contour *Use around the hairline of the forehead, in the hollows of the cheeks, and under the chin a little bit before the neck.*

Highlighter *Use above the apples of the cheeks.*

Blush *Use on the apples of cheeks and along the cheekbones, but not too low.*

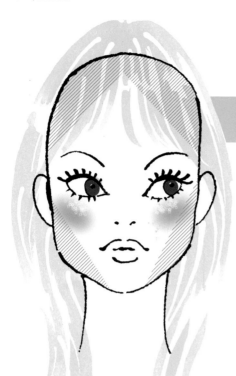

SQUARE FACE *These techniques soften the hard edges.*

Contour *Use on both side "corners" of the jawbone and the corners of the forehead, creating a diamond shape.*

Highlighter *Use above the apples of the cheeks.*

Blush *Use along the cheekbones.*

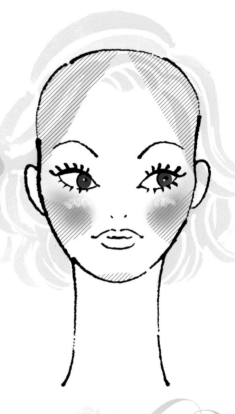

HEART-SHAPED FACE *The clever application of makeup will balance out the width of the forehead.*

Contour *Use at the temples and the sides of the forehead, and on the tip of the chin.*

Highlighter *Use above the apples of the cheeks.*

Blush *Start at the apples of the cheeks and blend back up to the temples.*

simple face shaping

I have two shaping methods for my face: one for every day, and one for special occasions. My everyday technique won't make you look five pounds thinner or banish the bloat that came with last night's sodium-laden sushi and soy-sauce dinner, but it will draw attention to your best features and even-out the rest.

■ NOSE JOB ON THE CHEAP ■

I have a nariz de bolla: a totally undefined and round nose. Here are two tricks I learned that will make you look like you had the nose job of your dreams: use a highlighter on the tip of your nose to give the illusion of lifting and defining your nose. Then, lightly apply a matte brown powder on the lower nostrils. Blend well, and you will have an instant nose job without having to pay a gazillion pesos to a world-famous plastic surgeon.

getting the look: everyday shaping

The application steps are the same regardless of your face shape, but exact placement of the highlighters and contours should be adapted to your own shape as outlined in the preceding illustrations. The shaping powder I use everyday is Symmetry by MAC.

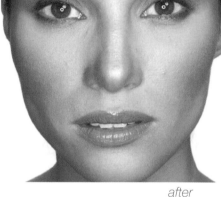

TOOLS:

✳ A medium, slightly angled applicator brush that covers a more targeted area.

✳ A loose matte brown contour concealer or matte bronzer.

✳ A lighter, luminescent highlighter cream.

✳ A large fluffy blending brush that covers a wide area.

✳ Loose translucent powder.

before   *after*

STEPS:

Use the concealer only where you have redness or discoloration. Use pointillism for any blemishes. The goal is to create an even-toned, fresh canvas for the defining powders without applying too much makeup beforehand.

✳ Using the medium, slightly angled applicator brush, apply the matte brown concealer lightly to your jawline, the hollows of your cheeks, your hairline, and the sides of your nose. Apply the darker concealer first because it requires the most blending.

✳ Using your fingertips, lightly apply the luminescent highlighter cream to the apples of your cheeks, down the center slope of your nose, and on your chin, the center of your forehead, and your eyelids.

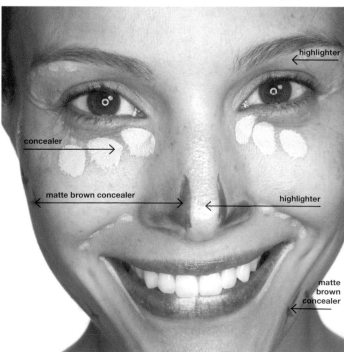

❋ Use a medium-size face brush to apply a very light coating of matte bronzer.

❋ Use the larger blending brush to apply a light coating of translucent loose powder to "seal" the makeup. To keep the skin dewy, apply the powder only to the under-eye area, the cheeks, the crease around the mouth, the chin, and the center of the forehead.

getting the look: shaping for special occasions

The goal is to make you look like a better version of yourself by defining the planes of your cheeks, chin, and temples. As with the everyday method, the application steps are the same regardless of your face's shape, but exact placement of the highlighters and contours should be adapted to your specific shape. This technique relies on creamy concealers instead of powder, because creamy concealers are more opaque and adhere to the skin better. I use this technique only for photo shoots and evening events. I recommend you do the same—trying to do this when you are in corre-corre mode is too much!

TOOLS:

❋ Yellow-based cream concealer two shades lighter than your own skin tone

❋ Brown cream concealer two or more shades darker than your skin tone

❋ Small blending sponge

STEPS:

❋ Start with a clean, moisturized face. If you need an under-eye concealer, apply it now. If you have very uneven skin tone, apply a thin layer of foundation.

❋ Using shorter strokes, apply the darker concealer to the areas you want to minimize according to your face shape.

❋ Apply a single swipe of the lighter concealer to the areas you want to bring to the foreground. For most women these are the cheekbones, the center of the nose, the chin, and possibly the center of the forehead.

❋ Dampen the makeup sponge with a quick spray of water. Squeeze out excess water.

❋ This step is where the artistry comes into play. Blend the concealer carefully and seamlessly into your face. Start by blending the darker areas and work into the lighter areas.

❋ Apply translucent powder to seal the makeup. Use a dry makeup sponge to apply powder only on the areas where you want to eliminate shine: under the eyes, the creases around the mouth, the chin, and the center of the forehead.

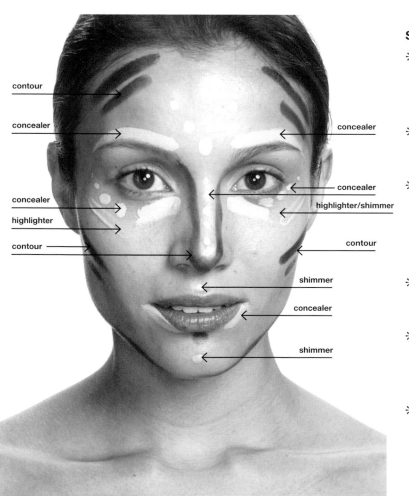

contour
concealer
concealer
highlighter
contour
concealer
highlighter/shimmer
concealer
contour
shimmer
concealer
shimmer

blush basics

After shaping your face, follow with your favorite blush on the apples of the cheeks. With so many different hues and formulas of blush available, many women find it difficult to choose a blush. We've all heard that we should choose a blush in a pinkish hue that matches the color our cheeks turn when your Tia Chole pinches them or when you come in from the cold, but I don't entirely agree. If you are like me, you probably want to minimize any redness on your skin. I have a touch of rosacea around my nose, which means I get a flush of red in that area. A pink or reddish blush would only make the discoloration look worse. So I stick to a tawny blush. You might find that a peachy hue is better, especially for everyday wear. I also recommend using a bronzer in place of blush. That said, a bright blush can create a really different look. When my face is clear, and even-toned, though, I love to play with bright colors on my cachetes. One of my favorite blushes is a bright pink by Anna Sui. See the chapter "Glamorama" for details, as well as ideas on how to choose a color palette depending on whether you want a strong or a subtle look. When I have my full red-carpet-ready face on—the foundation, the contour, the whole works—I break out the bright phosphorescent pinks that I love, because these pinks really pop!

As for formulas, here's a brief breakdown of the different types of blush on the market:

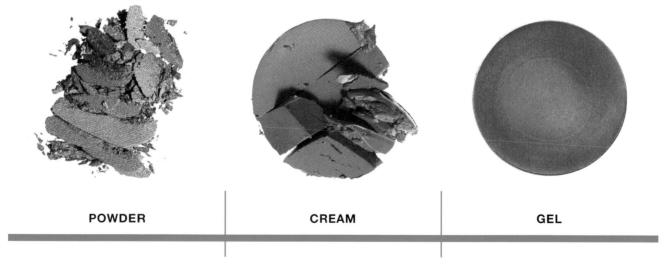

POWDER	**CREAM**	**GEL**
This is the most commonly used kind of blush; it's great for any skin type and is a must for the acne-prone, since gels and creams may clog pores.	This type of blush is great for dry skin; apply it before you apply loose powder.	This is harder to use because it dries so quickly that you have to work fast; gel should also be applied before you apply powder.

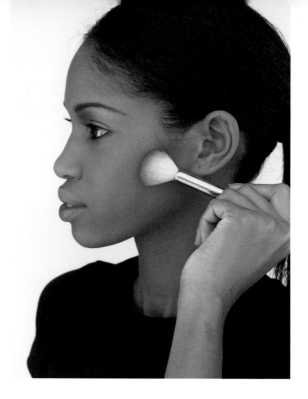

getting the look: powder blush

After you have applied foundation and completed shaping your face, finish with a light coating of translucent powder and then:

✳ Apply blush in a upward direction, starting on the apples of the cheeks and moving up and backward along the cheekbones.

✳ Blend well along the cheeks and into the shaded hollows below the cheekbone.

getting the look: cream or gel blush

After you have applied foundation and completed shaping your face, but before you have applied loose translucent powder:

✳ Dab a small amount of blush on the apples of the cheeks with your fingertips, blending upward and out toward the temples.

✳ If the color looks too faint, dab on a bit more blush and blend again. Build intensity gradually: it is much easier to apply more blush than to take it off after you have applied too much.

✳ Finish with a light coating of translucent powder.

bronzer, baby!

Bronzer is one of the greatest beauty weapons a girl can wield. It helps diminish redness, makes us look tanned and well rested, and enhances our features. Apply it wherever the sun naturally hits for a lasting glow. Here is a breakdown of the different formulas of bronzer:

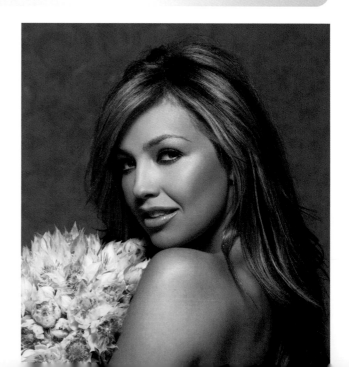

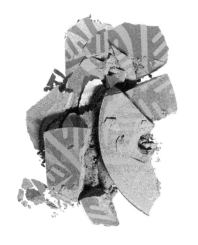

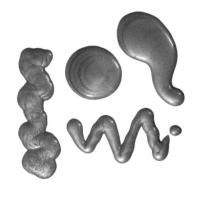

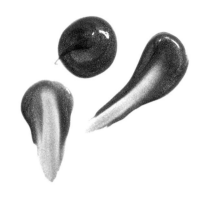

POWDER	GEL	LIQUID
This bronzer is easiest to apply. Use over your loose translucent powder.	Gel gives a dewy look, great for days spent outside. Like gel blush, it sets quickly, so be nimble with your fingertips when applying. For daily wear, I use a gel blush by Tarte. It gives a sporty glow.	This is slightly heavier than gel, so apply a little and build the color gradually. I typically use liquid bronzer on my body. My favorite is Flamingo Fancy by Benefit. It makes my piernas glow like a Victoria's Secret model's.

getting the look: powder bronzer

After you have applied foundation and completed shaping your face, finish with a light coating of powder and then:

❈ Apply bronzer with a fluffy blush brush anywhere the sun naturally hits the face: the cheeks, the forehead, the chin, and the nose.

❈ Blend well all over the face to eliminate lines of demarcation. The effect should be seamless.

getting the look: liquid or gel bronzer

After you have applied foundation and completed shaping your face, but before you have applied loose powder:

❈ Dab a small amount of bronzer with your fingertips where the sun naturally hits the face: cheeks, forehead, chin, nose.

❈ Blend well with fingertips. If the color looks too faint, dab on a bit more bronzer and blend again. Build intensity gradually: as with blush, it is much easier to apply more bronzer than to take it off after you have applied too much.

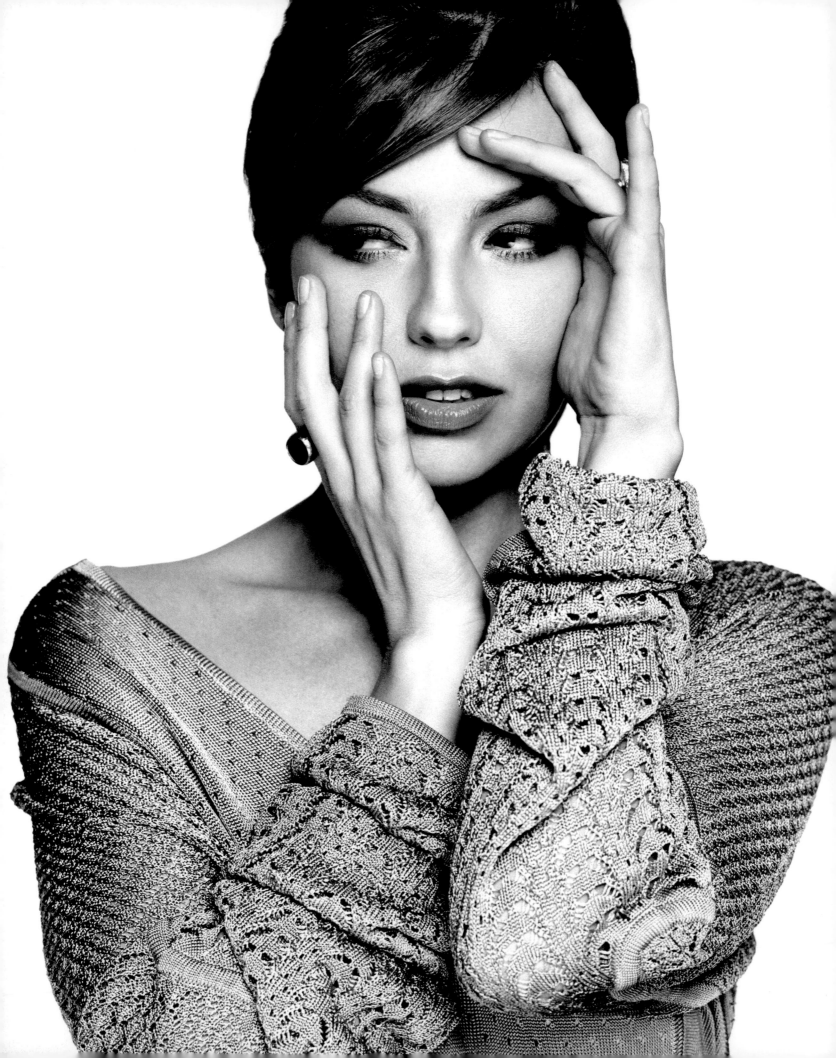

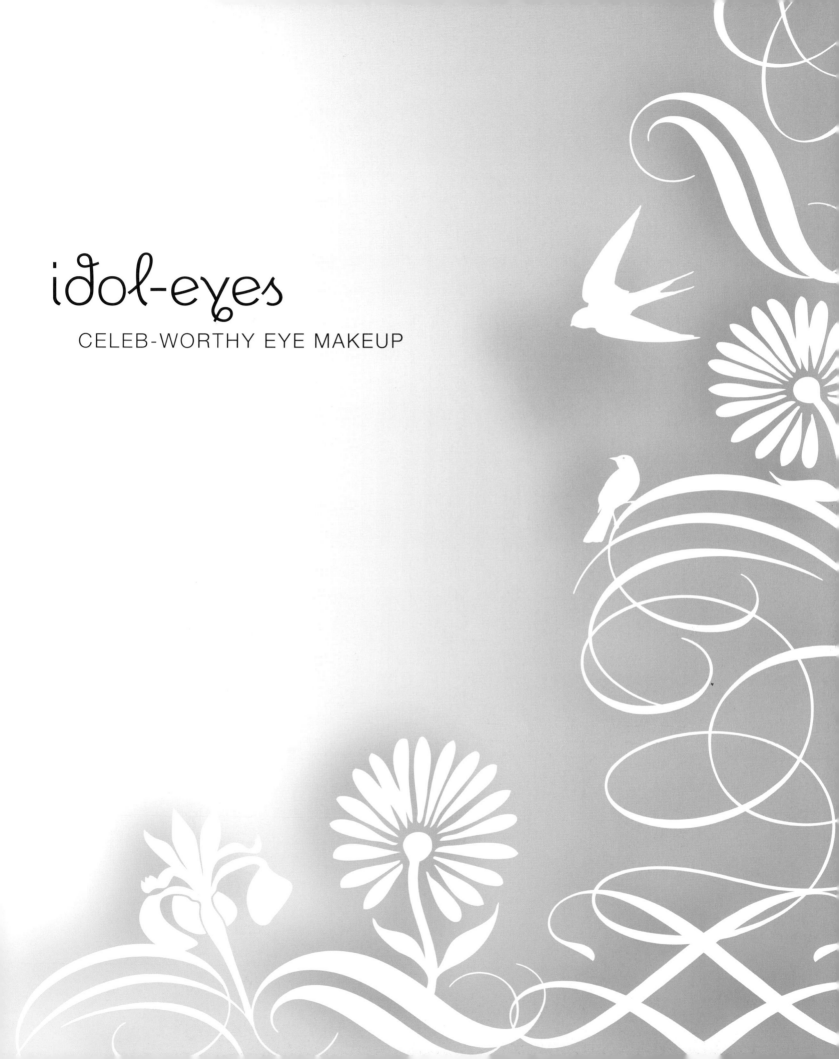

idol-eyes

CELEB-WORTHY EYE MAKEUP

Los ojos are the most expressive part of any woman's face—and the perfect place to add color and drama. Eye makeup can be bright and bold, smoky and sultry, sweet and flirty, or barely there. In this chapter I give you the goods on how to create multiple looks. First I'll show you the basics of brow shaping and grooming—there's much more to it than a pair of tweezers. Then we'll move on to the essentials of eye shadows, liners, and mascara.

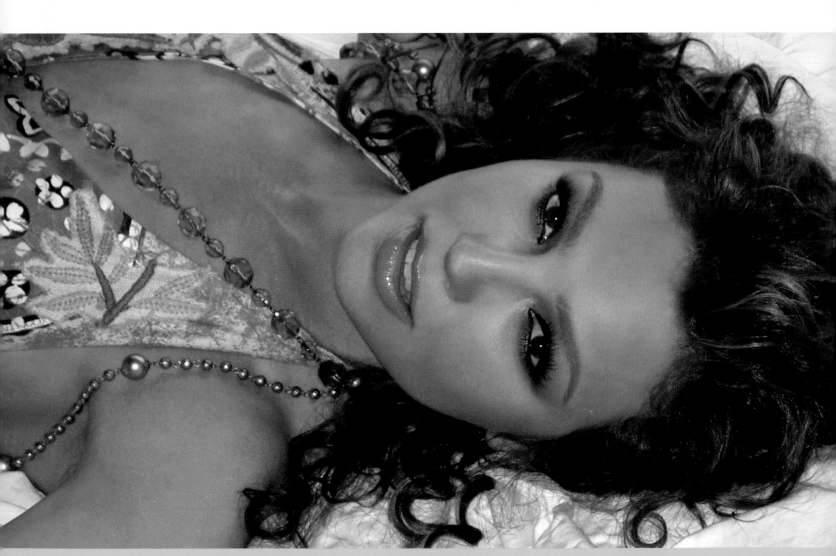

brow business

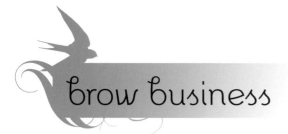

I'm a firm believer that eyebrows are the key to a finished, groomed look. They bring definition and balance to the features. For this reason, I knew I had to kick off the eye chapter by talking about eyebrows.

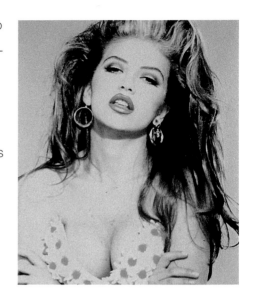

I am a fanatic about my brows. When I was younger, I let myself be convinced to try different looks with my brows, from a super-thick '80s mega brow to a pencil-thin mini brow. Not anymore. Even though I have access to the best makeup artists and aestheticians in the world, I do my own brows. It's true. I know what works for me and what makes me look my best. No waxing or threading for me. I use only tweezers, because they offer the most precision and control. But that's just me. Just because I have a DIY approach to plucking and primping doesn't mean that you need to do the same. If you are a brow-shaping virgin or feel like there is no way José that you are going to be able to tame and tweeze your monobrow into a pair of lovely cejitas, then by all means, get to an aesthetician. If you see someone with extraordinary brows, ask her where she got hers done. A great brow aesthetician is worth the investment.

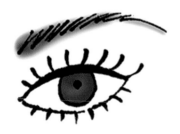

This illustration shows the optimal angles for where the brow should start and end, and where the natural arch tends to fall.

Before I get into the nitty-gritty, a word to the wise: the goal is not to pluck away your natural brow shape, but to clean up and streamline the brows you naturally have. I cannot stress this enough. Some women are lucky to have Brooke Shields eyebrows—they just need to tweeze, trim, and go. Others need a little boost to fill in empty spaces. As we age, our eyebrows do begin to thin out, which is why you might look at your mami one day and wonder where her eyebrows went. So before you wield those tweezers like a gardener on too much Red Bull, repeat this mantra: Better to undertweeze than to overpluck.

Different looks require different levels of maintenance. For every day, I simply apply brow gel to keep my eyebrows groomed. If I am going out, I'll use a light powder to give them a fuller, soft shape. When I am about to go onstage, I bring out the big guns: eyebrow pencils.

CELEB SECRET REVEALED!

During the summer, when I have a toasty (faux) tan going and my highlights are at their brightest, I use a colored brow gel—very light, almost gold in color—which creates a look as though I've bleached my brows. It's a beautiful soft look for summer.

getting the look: belissima brows

One of the most important tools for beautiful brows is an eyebrow pencil. To select the color, it is generally safer to go a few shades lighter than your brows—whether you are using pencil or powder. Lighter shades are more forgiving if you overdo it. Go heavy on too dark a color and you'll end up looking like Frida Kahlo—who was beautiful, but not everyone can pull off her look.

TOOLS:

❄ Tweezers

❄ Eyebrow brush, clean mascara brush, or fine-tooth comb

❄ Eyebrow pencil or eyebrow powder

❄ Brow gel

❄ Stiff-bristled eyebrow-powder brush

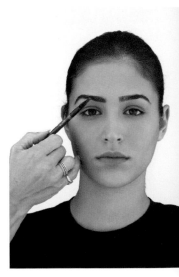

First, shape your brows.

❄ With the tweezers, start by plucking any stray hairs that fall outside your natural brow line. Pluck in the direction of the hair growth. Once you have removed the stray hairs, you are now trying to shape the brow along the brow's edge. Go one hair at a time.

❄ Repeat your mantra: Better to undertweeze than overpluck.

❄ One good guard against overplucking: work on each brow a little bit at a time. This helps you match one brow to the other.

❄ When you're finished plucking, use the brow brush, clean mascara brush, or fine-tooth comb to brush the brow hairs upward. This reveals gaps or areas of sparseness in the brows.

Fill in any bald spots or areas of sparse growth with the eyebrow pencil or brow powder.

If you are using pencil:

❄ Be sure the pencil has a nice sharp point.

❄ Use light, feathery strokes.

❄ If necessary, use spare strokes to extend the line of the brow. Extend the line slightly, or it will look obviously fake.

❄ Use the brow brush or a clean mascara brush to blend the pencil onto the brow. Again, brush upward. The end effect should be a more defined, yet not obviously drawn-in, brow.

❄ Seal the brows with brow gel.

If you are using powder:

❄ Apply it with a stiff-bristled eyebrow-powder brush after you have plucked and shaped the brows. Brow powder creates a softer line than brow pencil and is better for everyday and special occasion wear.

❄ Gently fill in the sparse areas; then, if you feel you need it, extend the line slightly.

❄ Use a brow brush to groom the brow hairs into place and blend in the powder.

❄ Finish with brow gel. Apply it sparingly, brushing the gel onto the hairs just enough to set the hair and seal the powder.

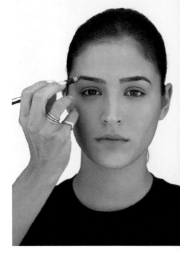

shady lady: apply eye shadow like a pro

I love eye shadow, because you can use it to create so many cool effects with so many different color options. To keep things simple, I'll start with a basic eye, then move on to some more daring looks.

getting the look: basic eye shadow

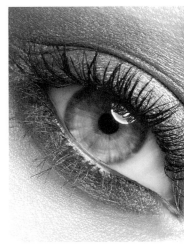

There are countless ways to apply eye shadow for myriad looks, but each one is built on one basic technique. Once you master it, you'll be ready to experiment with loads of different eye looks. In general, you'll want to use three shades, or tones, of eye-shadow color. Here is the full list of tools you'll need for ojitos coquetos:

✳ Eye-shadow base, which helps shadow to adhere and last longer. You can buy special cream bases specifically for eye shadow or simply use your regular foundation.

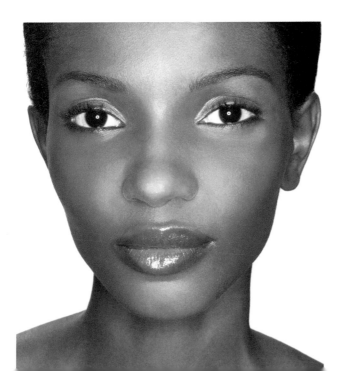

✳ All-over color, or lid color, in the medium of the three tones. This is the primary eye-shadow color; it is applied to the lid from the lash line to the brow line.

✳ Contour in a tone darker than the all-over color or lid color; this is used to reshape the eyes.

✳ Highlighter in the lightest tone of the three, for emphasis.

✳ Medium eye-shadow brush to apply the lid color and the highlighter.

✳ Small eye-shadow brush for creating contour and smoky eye effects.

With these tools in hand, you can create dreamy eyes. If you've never done it, following these steps may seem complicated, but don't worry: the technique takes no time to master.

✳ Using your fingertip, apply a light, oil-free foundation to the eyelid, or use an eye-shadow base to even out the skin tone. Apply a light dusting of translucent powder with your fingertip to set the base. Go easy with the powder: if you use too much, it will settle into the fine lines of the eye area, making them more noticeable.

✳ Brush on the lid color using the medium eye-shadow brush. Concentrate on the ball of the eye and brush from the lash line to the crease. If you are going for a very simple, groomed look, you can stop at this step and move on to the lashes.

✳ With the smaller contour brush, apply the darkest color along the crease. Begin from the inside and work outward.

✳ Blend the contour color well into the main lid color, using the medium brush.

✳ Switch back to the small contour brush. Apply the contour color along the bottom and top outside lash lines, as close to the lash line as possible.

✳ With the medium brush, apply the highlighter along the upper brow bone. Be careful not to apply too much, or it will make you look heavy-lidded.

learn your lines: pencil and liquid

I don't use eyeliner for everyday. For me, eye looks are all about experimentation. Sometimes I want a naked and romantic eye look, so I apply only mascara and a shiny nude shadow to my eyelid. Other times I want to look spicy and adventurous. Then I will use eye shadows and whip out my eye pencils, too. This is because nothing makes the eye pop like eyeliner. It makes the whites of your eyes look whiter and the shape of your eye more defined. Use a pencil for easier application. But for big events, try your hand at liquid liner, to get a Sophia Loren screen-siren look. Dark brown and black are the two most common eyeliner choices, because they define the eye and are almost mistake-proof colors. I think it is great to experiment with different color choices, though, and I'll show you how in the section on picking different color palettes. Whether you're using a pencil or liquid, apply eyeliner using a mirror in a well-lit area. Tilt the angle of the mirror so that you are looking down at the mirror and you can see your entire lid.

getting the look:
everyday eyes with penciled liner

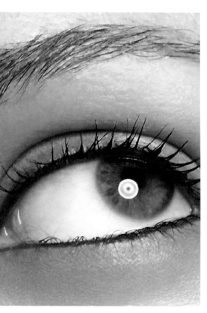

TOOLS:

✳ Eyeliner pencil

✳ Eyeliner pencil sharpener

✳ Q-tip or small, sponge-tip eye-shadow applicator

Always begin with a sharpened eye pencil. The tip of the pencil should be pointed, but soften the point slightly by rolling it in your fingertips.

✳ Pull your eyelid taut and begin at the inside corner, drawing little dots as close to the lash root as possible, each dot as close to the next as possible. Work from the inside outward.

✳ To make your eyes look bigger, slightly extend the liner beyond the outer edge of your eye. You can make this outside line slightly thicker for a more cat-eye look.

✳ To minimize any unevenness of line, use a Q-tip or sponge-tip applicator to soften and smoke the line of dots. I use an angled stiff-bristled brush to blend the line well with the roots.

✳ Line the lower lash line using careful, small strokes as close to the lash line as possible. On most women, eyeliner on the lower lid looks best when applied only on the outer two-thirds of the eye. The exception is when you are creating a dramatic, smoky eye. Then you want to apply your liner—pencil or powder—generously and around the entire eye or even on the inner rim.

■ **CELEB SECRET REVEALED!** ■

Pencil eyeliners are made of wax, which can melt. To avoid racoon eyes, "seal" the eyeliner—use a stiff angled brush to apply the same color eye shadow on top of the eyeliner.

getting the look: sexy, smoky eyes with liquid liner

Liquid and powder eyeliner combined make a potent and irresistible smoky eye combination.

TOOLS:

❋ Liquid eyeliner

❋ Stiff-bristled eyeliner-powder brush

❋ Powder eye shadow, powder eyeliner, or eyebrow powder

This technique takes a lot of practice, but the effect is amazing-sísimo! You'll get dark, flashing eyes worthy of a romantic evening or the red carpet.

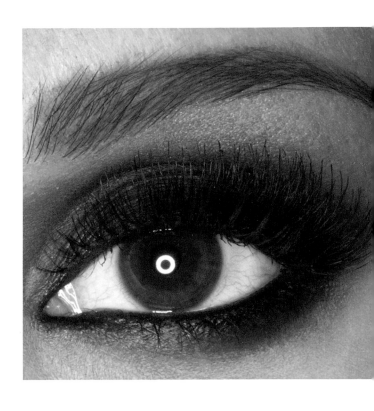

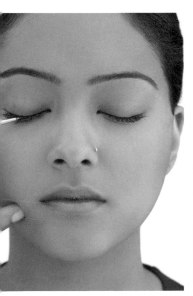
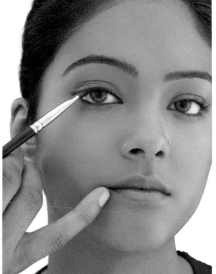

❋ Use one hand to pull the eyelid taut.

❋ With your other hand, brush with the liquid liner along the roots of the lashes from the inside out, as close to the lash line as you can possibly get. Hold steady!

❋ I've never seen anyone attempt to apply liquid liner on the lower lid and actually look good. Liquid liner is just too hard. Save that for the pencil or powder liner.

❋ Use the eyeliner-powder brush with dark eye shadow, eyebrow powder, or eyeliner powder to create a soft line directly on top of and slightly above the liquid line. Blend and extend the line to the outside edges of the eye for a smoldering cat-eye effect.

█ CELEB SECRET REVEALED! █

I am the Speedy Gonzales of makeup application. I need only five minutes to get ready. Since I live in fast-forward mode, I'm an expert at getting ready in a moving vehicle. What's the trick? Anchor your hand on your pinky! As you are applying mascara or eyeliner, for example, hold the wand or the pencil with your thumb, index, and middle finger, while your pinky is anchored on your cheek. ¡Arriba! ¡Arriba! ¡Andale!

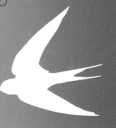

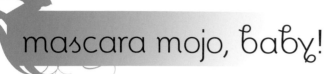

mascara mojo, baby!

Mascara is the icing on the cake—it lengthens, thickens, and darkens the lashes all at once, creating a beautiful frame for your stunning ojos. I recommend black mascara or dark brown, unless you are very fair haired and actually have blond lashes, in which case I would use a lighter color.

getting the look: thick lashes

TOOLS:

❋ Eyelash curler

❋ Eyelash primer (optional)

❋ Mascara

❋ Eyelash or eyebrow comb

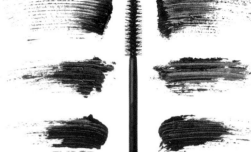

Now is the time to conquer all your fears of that intimidating contraption, the eyelash curler.

❋ Wield that eyelash curler like a ninja warrior: fearlessly and expertly place the rubber-edged bottom of the curler near the roots of your top lash line, clamp down slowly, and hold for five seconds. You won't feel a thing.

❋ I also do an extra clamp mid-lash so my lashes look curly instead of simply crimped.

❋ This is an optional step. Apply the white primer to the outer lashes, to extend them and give them more heft. Concentrate on the tips if you want to lengthen, or apply the primer to the entire lash to thicken. Let dry for thirty seconds.

❋ Before applying mascara, make sure there is no excess mascara on the wand. A good-quality mascara should have just enough deposited on the bristles. My favorites are Definicíls by Lancôme and Yves Saint Laurent's Infini

Curl Mascara. If your wand has too much, use a tissue to blot off the excess.

❋ Sweep the first layer of mascara outward from the roots of the upper lashes to the tips.

❋ The second and third applications should concentrate on the tips. Use the brush to build the mascara on the tips only, creating super-long-looking lashes.

❋ Wait about thirty seconds or so for the lashes to dry.

❋ Use an eyelash or eyebrow comb to smooth away any clumps.

❋ Wipe any excess mascara off the wand with a tissue. Then dab at your lower lashes with the tip of the wand to apply mascara to your lower lashes.

▰ CELEB SECRET REVEALED! ▰

I suffer from under-eye puffiness, especially when I don't get enough sleep. I take raw potatoes from the fridge (because they should be nice and cool), slice them, and place the slices on my eyes for fifteen minutes. It brings down all my puffiness, no matter how little sleep I've had. ¡Y listo!

faux lashes

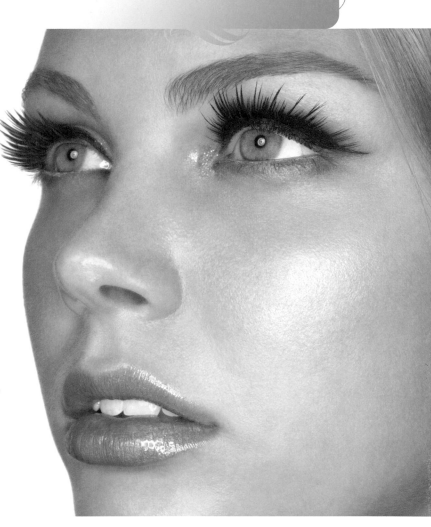

Falsies: I love them! I think in a former life I must have been a drag queen, because I adore the drama that false lashes create. My favorite types are the individual bunches of lashes that you can place strategically along your own lash line, and those fabulous, full eyelash strips made of mink. Mink eyelashes are a glossy deep auburn color. The effect they have: ¡Estupenda! It makes you look as if you have natural, full lashes that don't need mascara.

Don't lose your courage when faced with false lashes and glue. Like everything else, they just take practice, and I've simplified the process as much as possible. Put on false eyelashes after you have applied shadow and eyeliner, but before your mascara.

getting the look: false lashes

TOOLS:

✻ Eyelash glue

✻ A row of lashes for each eye, trimmed to fit the outer two-thirds of your lash line

✻ Tweezers

✻ Liquid liner (if necessary)

✻ Mascara

Set yourself up in a well-lit room, and keep a steady hand.

✻ Apply glue to the bottom edge of a lash strip. Wait thirty seconds, until the glue is slightly tacky to the touch.

✻ Using the tweezers, pick up the lashes as close to the strip as possible and carefully place the strip as close as you can to the lash line on the outer two-thirds of the eye. Gently use the tweezers to apply slight pressure until the glue "holds." If you are nimble enough, use your fingers instead of tweezers.

✻ Wait at least thirty seconds for the glue to set. The ends of the strip must adhere for long-lasting hold. If needed, use black or dark brown liquid liner to gently cover any telltale "seams."

✻ Apply a light coat of mascara to blend your natural lashes with the fake ones.

shape shifting: special effects for eyes

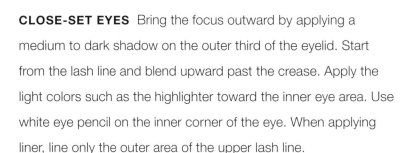

SMALL EYES To create the illusion of larger eyes, choose a contour color only slightly darker than the lid color, instead of the high-contrast mix you usually use. Apply it only to the outer two-thirds of the crease, above the ball of the lid. If you wear eyeliner, avoid lining the entire lash line with a dark color, because that would have a closing effect on the eyes.

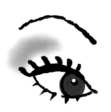 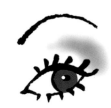

CLOSE-SET EYES Bring the focus outward by applying a medium to dark shadow on the outer third of the eyelid. Start from the lash line and blend upward past the crease. Apply the light colors such as the highlighter toward the inner eye area. Use white eye pencil on the inner corner of the eye. When applying liner, line only the outer area of the upper lash line.

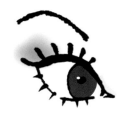 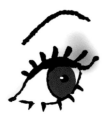

WIDE-SET EYES Here you do the opposite of the technique for close-set eyes. Apply the darker contour color in the inner eye area, from the inner corner up past the crease toward, but not reaching, the inner brow line.

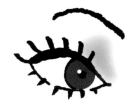 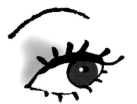

ROUND EYES To create the illusion of more almond-shaped eyes, apply a contour color to the outer area of the lids. Line only the outer top lash line, because bottom eyeliner will accentuate the roundness of the eye shape.

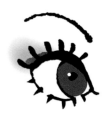 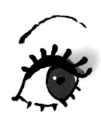

▪ LASH LESSONS

I've read endless tips on makeup-bag must-haves for special nights out. Here is one secretito that you will read only here: if you are going to wear false eyelashes, take your eyelash glue with you! I learned the hard way—at a gala with photographers absolutely everywhere. Everyone was looking their best, having a great time, and there I was, trying to smile for the cameras while hoping no one noticed that my lash line was suddenly askew. Not a fun way to spend a glamorous, fabulous night out on the town, believe me.

¡eye-yayai!

Here is where we start to have fun. I created these different eye looks to encourage you to break out from the same old humdrum lid color, contour, and highlighter combo you always use. Grab your makeup kit and try these eye looks!

brigitte bardot eyes

This look mimics the dramatic eyes of the 1960s.

✳ Start by preparing the eye with an eye-shadow base, to even out discoloration on the lid and create a base that will help the eye makeup adhere.

✳ Apply a matte white color to the entire lid using a medium eye-shadow brush, beginning at the lash line and extending up toward your brow.

✳ Using a grey matte eye-shadow and a small eye-shadow brush, apply the shadow along the crease of your eye to contour. Start from the inner eye and work outward. Make the line slightly wider as you approach your outer eye, but then taper to a fine point as you extend the line.

✳ Don't blend! The idea here is to be bold and exaggerated.

✳ Next is the eyeliner. Use sharp, black eyeliner to line your entire upper lid along the lash line or use liquid—whichever is easier.

✳ Extend the line outward and upward beyond your lash line. Make the line slightly thicker as it goes toward the outer edge of your eye.

✳ Use white eyeliner to line the inner rim of your eye. This will make the whites of your eyes look larger and whiter.

✳ This eye look demands false eyelashes! Apply a strip along the top lashes.

✳ Use a black eye pencil or liquid liner to cover any excess eyelash glue.

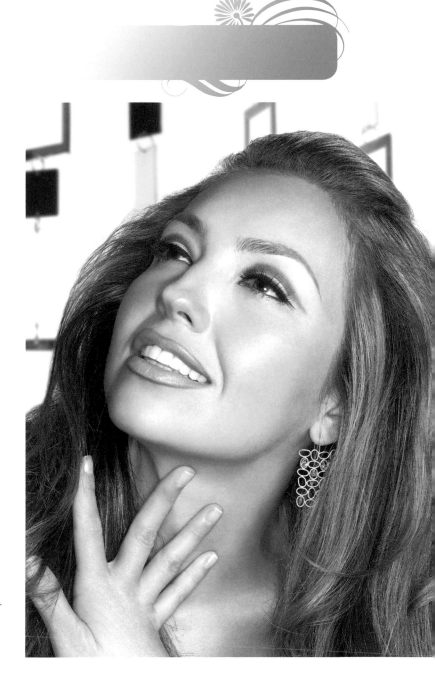

✳ Apply a generous coat of black mascara to the top lashes.

✳ Apply a generous coat of mascara to the bottom lashes too, creating that doll-like, wide-eyed look typical of the '60s.

✳ The eyes are so strong here, keep the rest of your makeup as simple as possible.

✳ Make sure brows are perfectly groomed, as the eyes here are the focus of the face.

peacock-pretty eyes

This beautiful look was inspired by the bright, saturated colors of the peacock feather.

❋ Prepare the eye with an eye-shadow base or a concealer to even out discoloration and ensure the eye color will hold.

❋ Start with a shimmery golden eye shadow and apply it to the entire eyelid with the medium eye-shadow brush, from the lash line to the eyebrow, especially to highlight the brow bone.

❋ Use a small eye-shadow brush to begin applying the strong, iridescent green to the ball of the eyelid. Apply in layers, deepening the color with each application.

❋ Extend the color to the crease and slightly above, stopping at the beginning of the brow bone.

❋ Use the small eye-shadow brush to apply a navy blue eye shadow along the entire bottom lash line. This is a colorful smoky eye, so as you did with the top lid, apply the shadow in layers, deepening the color with each application.

❋ Apply the shimmery gold to the inner corners of the eye and blend outward.

❋ Use clear eyelash glue to adhere a strip of false lashes to the top lash line.

❋ Apply several coats of black mascara to the lashes.

❋ Continuing with the golden-hued tones, use a bronzing cheek color and a simple pearlescent gloss to finish the face.

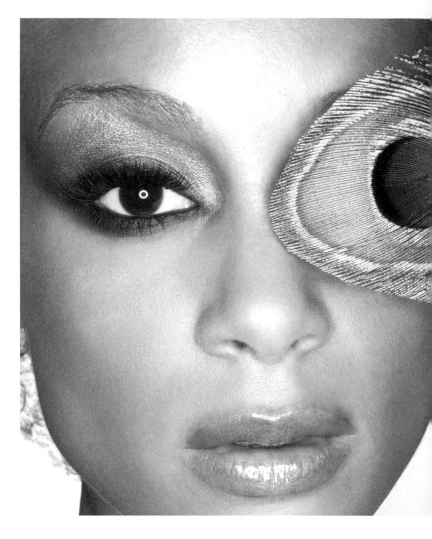

taking the red-eye

Here is an edgy eye look that is meant to be different and experimental.

✳ Prepare the eyelid area with eye-shadow base.

✳ Use a medium eye-shadow brush to apply a blood-red matte shadow in the inner corner of the eye and on the ball of the lid.

✳ Use a small eye-shadow brush to line the top lash line and the outer bottom lash line with matte purple eye shadow.

✳ Blend the two colors seamlessly along the top lash line with the small eye-shadow brush, so you can't tell where one color ends and the other begins.

✳ Apply white shimmer underneath the eyebrow arch.

✳ Curl the lashes and coat with an application of mascara.

✳ Keep the rest of your makeup simple: a wash of color on the cheeks and a clear, no-color gloss on the lips for high shine.

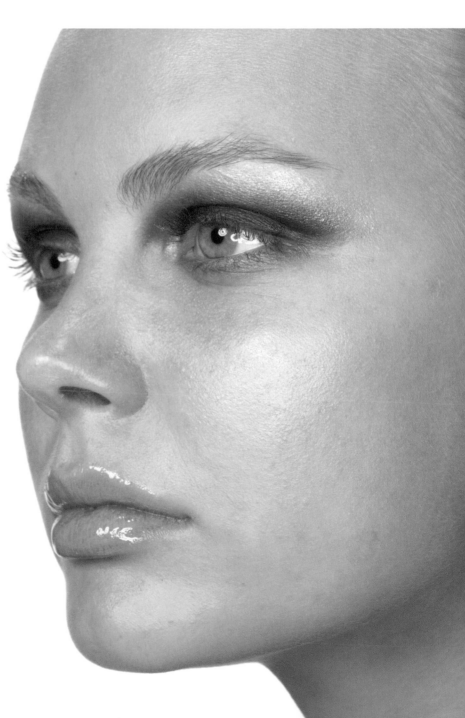

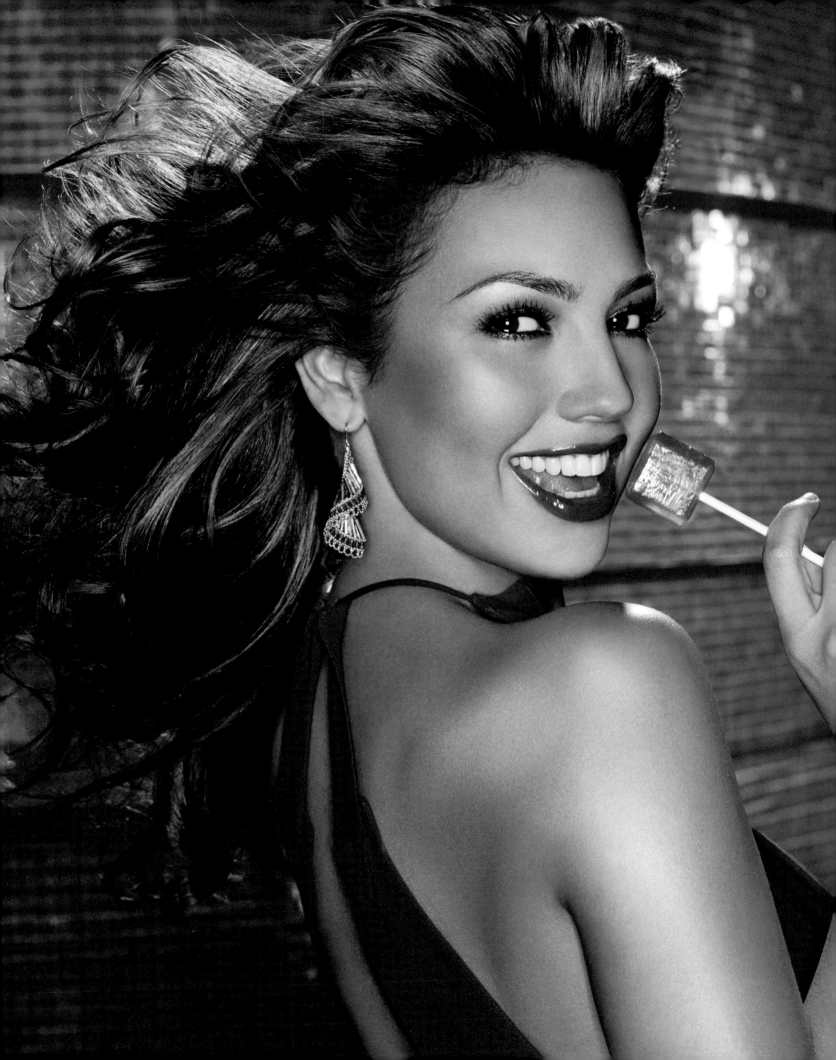

luxe lips

THE BEST CARE AND COLOR

I was once included on a list of "prettiest smiles" in one of those weekly celebrity mags. Halle Berry was one of the other celebrities chosen. Needless to say, I was very flattered. Being happy and at peace are key to a great smile, but give a girl the right gloss, and her grin will go from simply sweet to super stunning—even on her off days.

In our collagen-injected world, I still believe that nothing makes a sonrisa sizzle like lip gloss. The right color can brighten up your whole face and give you an easy glow. Lip gloss is perfect for everyday wear. Still, I do reach for my lip-liner and lipstick especially, when I am performing onstage and need smudge-proof color that won't fade away by my third song. There are so many different looks you can achieve by combining different products and techniques, it's no wonder that most women have more lip colors in their makeup bags than any other cosmetics item.

prepainting prep

The skin on your lips needs extra care, because your lips have no oil-producing glands. This leaves them prone to chapping and fine lines. Here's how I pamper my pucker:

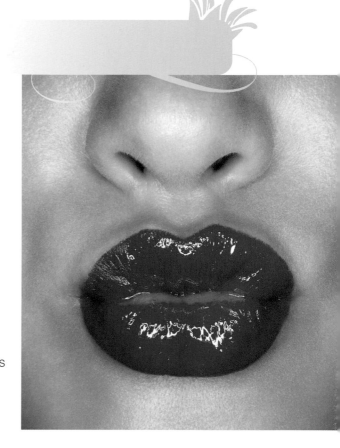

✳ Use a soft toothbrush or the rough side of a washcloth to gently exfoliate the lips in your daily shower.

✳ Apply thick lip balm after you get out of the shower, to keep the lips hydrated.

✳ New exfoliating lip creams help diminish the thin lines that develop on the lip line, while keeping the lips moisturized. One of my favorites is Neostrata AHA Lip Conditioner.

✳ At night, apply lip cream or a thick balm before going to bed.

lip lessons

Prepping the lips gives you a soft surface for whatever lip color and lip formula you are going to apply. Because the formulas and their effects differ dramatically, the application technique depends on what kind of product you use. The choices for lip color are also widely varied. Here is a quick breakdown of which formula is best for which look.

Matte Best for deep, rich color with a very defined lip line; matte is not good for very dry lips. Apply over lip-liner with a lip brush— it is much more precise. Begin applying it at the center of the lip and work outward to the edge of the lip line.

Cream Best for rich color with more moisturizing properties. As with the matte formula, apply cream lip color with a lip brush over lip-liner. Begin applying it at the center of the lip and work outward to the edge of the lip line.

Sheer Best for a fresh, simple wash of color, especially during the day. Apply it without first using a lip-liner. Use a lip brush, or even your finger. Blot the lips on a tissue for a subtle stained look.

Gloss Best for a high shine with varying degrees of pigment. Apply it with the doe-foot applicator that comes with most glosses, a tiny lip brush, or even your fingertip. In general, the lighter the texture, the easier gloss is to apply.

Stain Best for a wash of color that is long-lasting, yet still light and subtle. A heavy kissing session will leave no evidence on your kissee. Don't apply it with your finger, because lip stains do leave pigment behind! Use the applicator that comes with the lip stain. When in doubt, use a Q-tip. Stains, unfortunately, do tend to dry the lips.

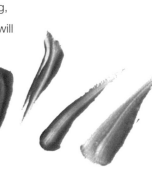

lip-liner application basics

Lip pencils create a base for lip color to adhere to, plus they leave a lasting tint that, unlike your lip color, will stick around long after lunch and coffee. I'm a big fan of using lip-liner in a shade that most closely matches the natural color of your own lips. This allows you to use the same pencil for many different lip colors, avoiding the dreaded "but does the lip-liner match my lipstick?" worry that is such a waste of time. The exceptions to this rule are certain types of reds, but we will get into that later. To properly apply lip-liner:

❋ Make sure that lips are exfoliated and soft. Apply a little lip balm or ChapStick so lips won't get too dry.

❋ Draw a thin line along the edge of your lips with sharpened lip-liner.

❋ If you don't have a steady hand or worry you might stray from your natural lip line, use the connect-the-dots technique: apply the lip-liner along the edge of the lip line in short, feathery strokes, as close together as possible.

❋ Then take the pencil and connect the dots to form an even line.

❋ Fill in the lips with the lip-liner for a longer lasting wear.

▬ CELEB SECRET REVEALED! ▬

Celine Dion gave me some excellent advice on how to avoid the dreaded hair-that-gets-stuck-in-your-lip-gloss-in-front-of-the-photographers-on-the-red-carpet-leaving-you-with-gloss-stains-on-your-face moment: Check the direction of the wind before you step outside. Right there, in your limo, when the door is opened and you are about to step out, use your hand to check the direction of the wind, then extract yourself so that your face is toward the wind. So what if your back is to the photographers? Just wait until the breeze changes. Then twirl around, smiling as big as you can, still fabulous, with your lips hair-free. The same holds for everyday encounters, too: If you feel a breeze coming on, turn your face to the wind. Another option: use a lip stain with ChapStick on top instead of lip gloss, which will make your lips less shiny but will still keep them supple. No more gloss marks on your face from hair that got stuck.

shape shifting: special effects for lips

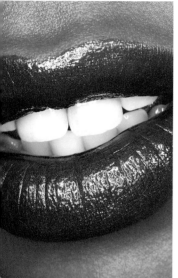

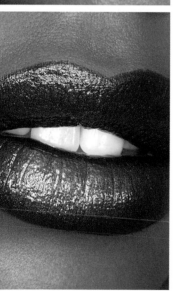

No one's boquita is perfect, unless she is Scarlett Johansson. And even she probably has some lip tricks up her sleeve. With the tricks and techniques here, you can use lip color to transform your lips to near perfection.

UNEVEN LIP TONE   Some Latinas tend to have uneven pigment in their lips. Following are two solutions.

❋ Find a lip-liner that matches the color of the darker lip area. Line and fill in the lips with this lip-liner before applying color.

❋ Or, apply sheer foundation as a primer. It will even out any discoloration, and it gives the lipstick something to adhere to.

THIN LIPS   Use lip-liner to accentuate your lip shape and make your lips look fuller.

❋ Use a lip-liner whose color is as close to your own lip tone as possible. Draw along the line where your lips and skin meet, not on the skin itself.

❋ Use a clean lip brush to blend the liner slightly inward. This "builds" the natural lip line ever so subtly.

❋ Avoid dark and matte colors. Opt for light, high-shine, and high-shimmer glosses.

UNEVEN LIP SHAPE   Use lip-liner to define a new shape.

❋ As with thin lips, use a lip-liner whose color is as close to your own lip tone as possible. Draw slightly above the edge of the lip line on the thinner part of the lip.

▦ WRINKLE RESCUE ▦

Hate those fine lines that develop around the lips as we age? There is no miracle cure in a bottle (I'll be the first to let you know when that goes on sale!), but you can take some steps to minimize the lines and even delay those suckers from showing up.

Don't smoke. Not only does cigarette smoke unleash an icky aging free-radical assault on your skin and leave you with bad breath and yellow teeth, the very action of puckering up and taking a puff repeatedly will make those tiny lines appear faster and deeper than if you were a nonsmoker. Puckering should be for kissing only!

Use a lip exfoliating cream that both removes dead skin and helps plump up the skin around the lips. Keeping the lips and their surrounding skin hydrated is key to minimizing the appearance of fine lines.

Try one of the new reverse lip-liners on the market. These are colorless matte lip-liner pencils that you apply directly outside the lip line. The pencils lock lip color on the lips and prevent creepage. DuWop makes one called Reverse Lipliner, and Mally Beauty makes one called Lip Fence.

And if the damage is too advanced: laser resurfacing, baby! I'll go over this in the "Extreme Beauty" chapter.

❋ Draw on the inner edge of the lip line on the thicker part of the lip.

❋ Blend the line inward, and brush on lip color inside of the lip-liner.

THICK LIPS Women are currently paying hundreds of dollars to plump their lips, but if you feel you have too much of a good thing, try the following.

❋ Cover your lips lightly with foundation.

❋ Using a lip-liner in a color that closely matches your skin tone, outline just inside the natural line of the lips.

❋ Apply color inside the lip-liner. Avoid high-shine and shimmering formulas.

pump up your pout

In Mexico, girls rub jalapeños on their lips to really get a bee-stung, flushed, and pouty look for their *labios*. Trust me: there are much less painful ways to plump up your kisser.

PLUMPING FORMULA GLOSS OR PRIMER Most plumpers on the market bring a flush to the lips that is alluring. I don't use these for daily wear, but for a hot date or special occasion, they can't hurt. My personal pick is Lip Venom by DuWop.

HIGHLIGHTER Apply a lip highlighter on the bow of the upper lip—the area where the two humps of the upper lip meet—and along the outside edges of the lower lip. This creates a frame that gives just the tiniest illusion of fullness. I recently bought a set of lip highlighter pencils called Flawless Fix Pencil by Laura Mercier. They come in light pink to skin-tone colors and are meant to be used to highlight the top and the bottom of the lip. They also help keep lip color in place. ¡Me encanta!

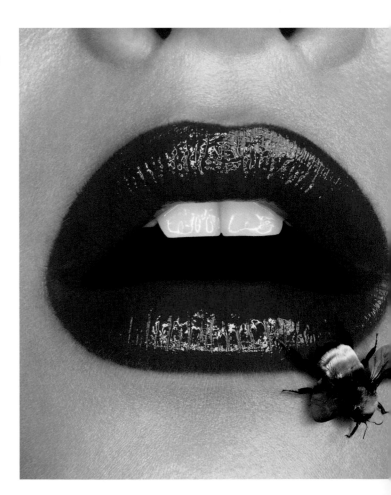

CONCEALER Apply a concealer a shade lighter than your own skin tone to the lips to brighten them, draw light, and give the illusion of plumpness. Concealer also works as a base for your lip color. Simply apply the concealer with your fingertips, blend well, and then apply your normal lip color and lip-liner over the lips.

LIP-LINER Your best tool for slightly building the lip line, and for adding a tiny layer to the lips by filling them in after you have outlined, is lip-liner.

GOLD IRIDESCENT LIP-LINER Applied slightly outside the lip line, this liner brings a shine to the lips for a popping effect, which also gives better definition to the mouth. Be cautious with this technique: the line should not be too obvious. Soften the line with a Q-tip after you apply it.

SHIMMER FORMULAS Avoid flat or matte formulas for your lip color. These dull your lips' natural curves and dimensions. Select shimmery formulas and, when in doubt, use light colors rather than dark ones.

GLOSS Right in the middle of your pucker is sweet spot for gloss. Apply ultra-high-shine gloss over your color to give your lips a visual boost.

MATTE BROWN POWDER A little dot of matte brown right under the fullest part of your bottom lip creates a visual illusion: since the skin under the lip appears to recede, your own natural lip appears fuller. Apply it sparingly and blend it well into the surrounding skin.

righteous rojo

It's a stereotype: the fiery, hot, spicy Latina with bright red lipstick, swaying her hips and doing the cha-cha. I don't like stereotypes, but I love red lipstick. I especially love bright electric coral red, which looks youthful. Wine matte red is also a classic look that can't go wrong.

It's essential to find the right red hue for your skin tone. One of the makeup artists I work with makes his own reds for the different clients he works with. For instance, he personally mixes a red for Angelina Jolie that makes her lips look flushed and stained instead of a severe, harsh red. He mixes reds on the movie or video set, using old-school formulas such as matte or cream to tailor the red and make a woman look her best. Try mixing the reds you have on hand—you might come up with a gorgeous shade just right for you. If mixing the perfect red seems intimidating and you'd rather use just one color, stick to a blue-red or brown-red formula, because orange-based red can be tricky: it's difficult to match the right shade to your skin tone, and it can emphasize any blotchiness in the skin. Still doubtful? Opt for a red in a gloss formula, which will give you a pop of color without the commitment of traditional red lipstick.

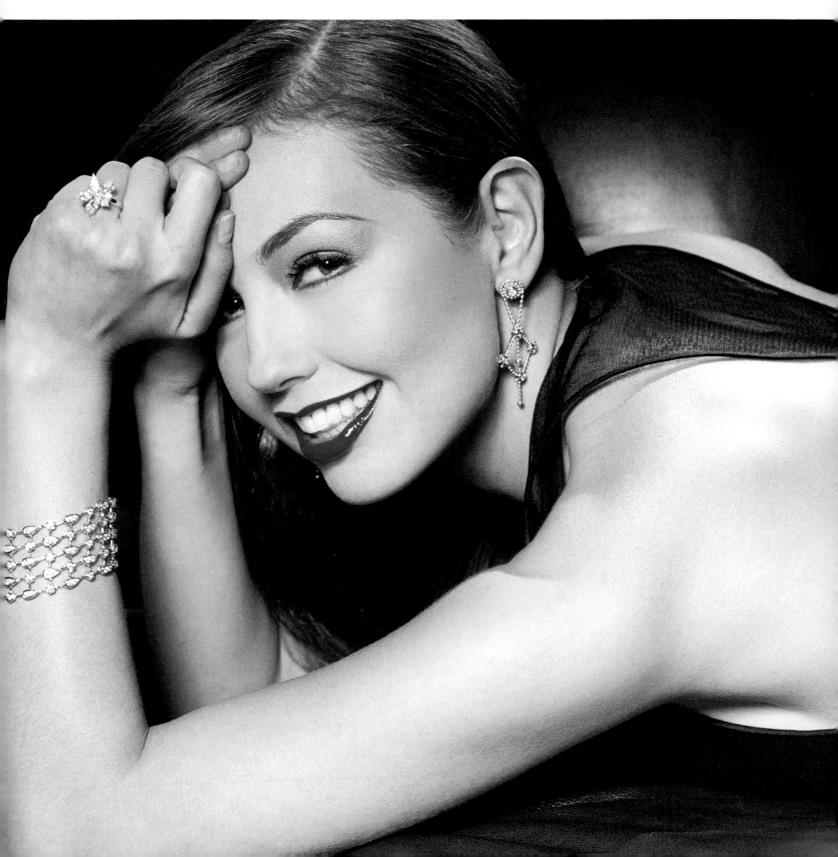

getting the look: racy red lips

Applying red lipstick is an art. No matter which red you ultimately choose, follow these simple steps.

TOOLS:

❋ ChapStick or nongreasy lip balm

❋ Lip plumper (optional)

❋ Nude-toned lip-liner

❋ Lip brush

❋ Creamy or matte red lip color

❋ One-ply tissue (regular tissue with the two sheets taken apart)

❋ Loose powder (optional)

❋ Glittery gloss (optional)

Red lipstick should be applied only on well-hydrated lips with no excess dry skin.

❋ Prepare the lips by exfoliating them and applying ChapStick or another wax-based balm to keep the lips supple, but not sticky. Blot the lips. If you are going for a plumped pucker, apply some lip plumper now.

❋ Use a lip-liner that closely resembles your natural lip color to line and fill in the lips. This creates an even canvas for the lipstick.

❋ With the lip brush, apply the red lip color starting at the inside of the middle lower lip. Blend outward toward the lip line. Repeat with the upper lip, taking extra care not to color beyond the lip line.

❋ Use the tissue to gently blot off excess lip color. Creamy and matte lip colors have strong pigments in the formula, so excess product on your lips will simply increase any potential smudging or smearing—not make the lipstick last longer.

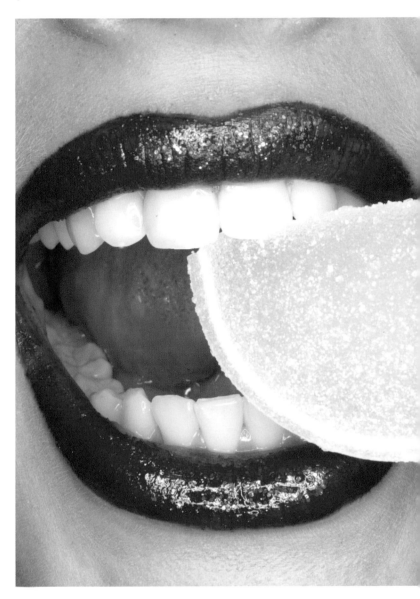

❋ For extra staying power, and if you do not tend to have dry lips, place the one-ply tissue on top of the lips and use the lip brush to apply loose powder over the tissue. A very thin coating of powder will remain on your lips, creating a matte look.

❋ Follow with a second coat of lipstick.

❋ To update the classic red lips, follow with a top coat of glittery gloss, like we did here.

lip-locking lessons

We Latinas tend to greet family and friends with kisses on the cheek, and celebrities have taken up this kissy-kissy greeting en masse. Europeans do it once on each cheek. Some of them even do it three times! But glossy girls have to take extra care to not leave a smear of their favorite lip color on their tías and girlfriends. And as for the men in our lives, they like lip gloss and lipstick when it's on us, not on them. So what do I do when I am about to greet and kiss the cheeks of a roomful of people, celebrities and family members alike? I do the cheek-to-cheek thing, with no lips involved. Touch the shoulders of the other person and give him or her a genuine hug so it won't look like you are being cold or frivolo. With your honey, leave the lip-kissing to later. Then be a sweetie and wipe off any residual lip color that might have migrated from your lips to his.

pearly brights

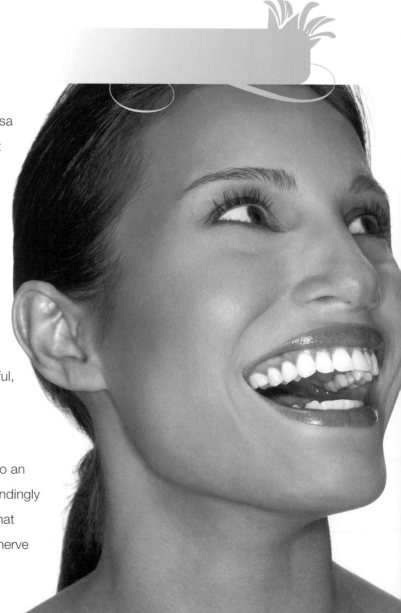

It's not enough to have gorgeous lips—for a fabulosa sonrisa you need straight, shiny choppers, too. Teeth are the latest area that beauty-obsessive women have begun to worry about. Believe me, I understand what it is like to avoid smiling because you don't like your teeth: I had braces when I was younger, and to this day I use Invisalign clear braces to help retain my teeth in the position I suffered to put them in via many trips to the orthodontist. In keeping with my Howard Hughes–like tendencies, I always carry a travel-size teeth-care kit, and I brush and floss after every meal. Having clean, healthy teeth is vital to having a beautiful, kissable smile.

Another beauty obsession with teeth is whiteness. I tried a tooth-bleaching process in which my teeth were exposed to an extra-bright laser light for about an hour. They came out blindingly white, but after the treatment, my teeth were so sensitive that when a cold wind hit them, I could feel it right down to the nerve endings. And ever since, I have had to brush my teeth with toothpaste made especially for people with sensitive teeth. I would never put myself through that whitening process again. I have to be fair, though: I have friends who have tried the same process and had a much better experience. The lesson here is to find out as much as you can about the process before you undergo it. If you have a tendency toward sensitive teeth, be extra cautious. I have found that I do like Crest White Strips. If I have a big event, I use the white strips beforehand. They give a nice boost to the whiteness and shine of my smile.

CELEB SECRET REVEALED!

One smile killer to be wary of—besides spinach stuck between your two front teeth—is lipstick smeared on your teeth. My friend Ana Luisa Pelufo, a screen siren from the heyday of old Mexican cine de oro, taught me this foolproof trick to avoiding that pitfall: After you apply your final coat of lip color, stick your finger in your mouth and suck on it like it's a chupete. Pull the finger out of your mouth. Any excess lipstick or gloss that might have made its way to your teeth and marred your sunny sonrisa is now on your finger, where you can safely wipe it off with a tissue.

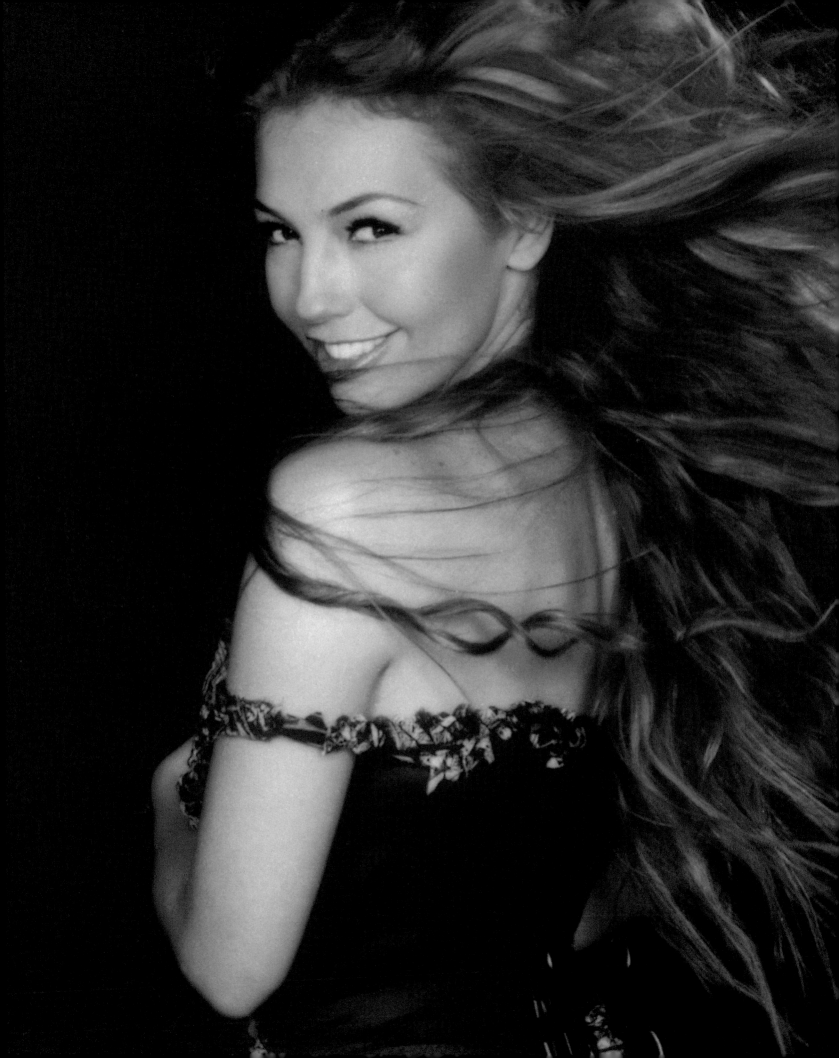

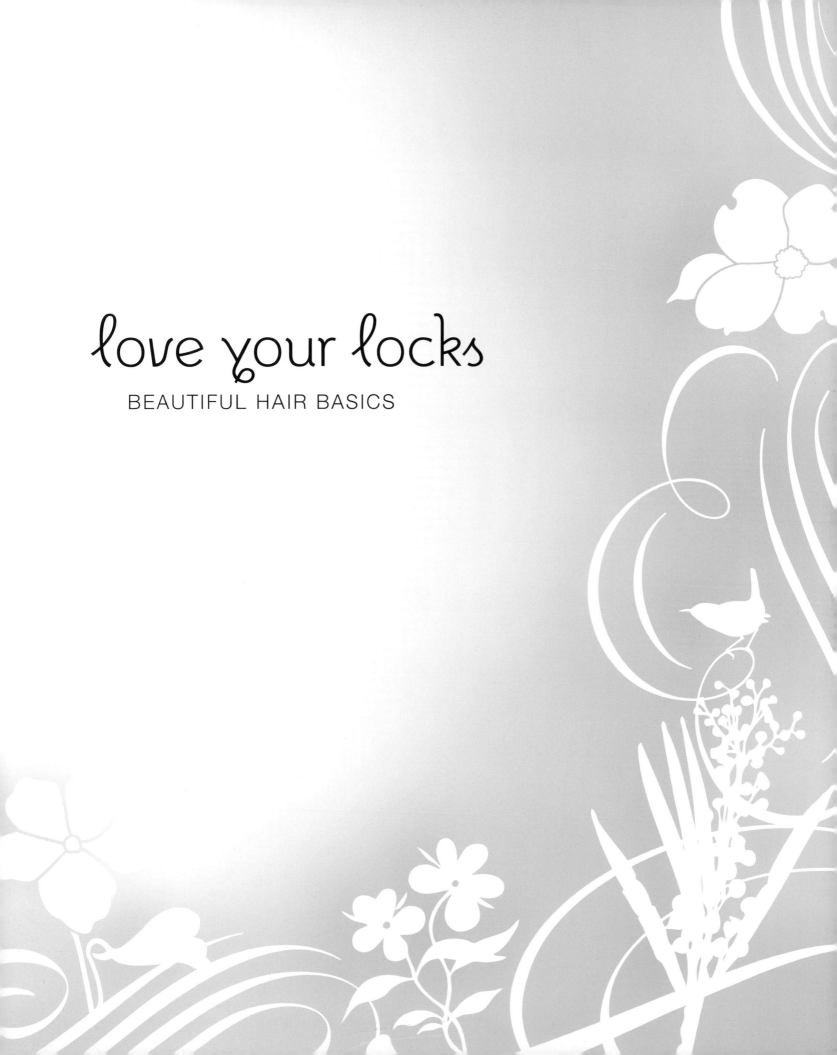

love your locks

BEAUTIFUL HAIR BASICS

You know that story about Samson and Delilah?

Where Samson is a big strong he-man, but the secret of his strength lies in his hair? When Delilah cuts it, Samson turns into a ninety-eight-pound weakling. I know a lot of women like Samson, myself included! We derive our strength and power from our hair. Our sex appeal, personality, and confidence are all tied up in our locks. That's a lot of pressure for a hairstyle!

To help you flex your Samson strength, I'm going to share all my secrets for a healthy mane. I've included styling tips for all hair types, whether your locks are long, short, straight, wavy, kinky, curly, or coarse. Ditch the ponytail rut by trying out a new style that works with your hair type. But before you even think about touching a blow-dryer, read on for ways to make your hair beautiful before it's styled. Hair reflects how you treat it from the inside out. A poor diet and bad lifestyle habits can put a damper on your 'do.

know your hair

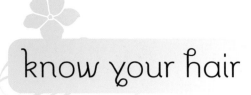
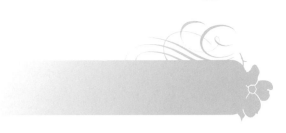

The outer layer of each strand of hair is called the cuticle, which is formed by tightly packed scales that overlap like shingles on a roof. If your hair is dull or prone to tangling and breakage, you might have damaged cuticles. Conditioning them is the first step to shiny, healthy hair. To smooth your cuticles, try a moisturizing conditioning treatment or protein-rich conditioners, which attempt to strengthen the overall hair shaft by boosting keratin (hair protein). One of my favorite hair masks is Nutritive Masquintense by Kerastase. I use it every four days to repair and protect my hair. Some other critical need-to-knows:

Stress affects your hair. In worst-case scenarios, it can lead to breakage and even bald spots! In general, though, if you make sure you get enough B vitamins through whole grains, yogurt, and oily fish such as salmon, your hair should be getting the basic nutrients it needs. If you have a demanding job or are going through stress in your life, try to add B vitamins to your diet via supplements or foods rich in these vitamins.

A diet of too little fat can make your hair dull and sin vida. Women who suffer from bulimia or anorexia wreak havoc on their hair by robbing their bodies of nutrients that are essential to healthy hair. Make sure you eat good-for-you fats from nuts and olive oil to promote a healthy shine.

Seasonal changes affect your hair and scalp just as they do your face and body. In the winter, besides becoming drier, your hair can be affected by static. Frequent heat styling can also affect hair health. I adjust my shampoo and conditioner to the time of year, using a richer conditioner in the winter and a lighter one in the summer.

Healthy hair grows about six inches a year, but split ends can travel up the hair strand quickly, undermining your attempts to grow your hair to a longer length. If you get regular trims, your ends will be less likely to split. I get my hair trimmed every two months and tell my stylist, "Cortame una pestañita de Barbie." That means "Cut only as much hair as Barbie's eyelash." That tiny bit keeps my growing hair healthy.

how to find the right hairstylist

I never let a crabby person near my mane with a pair of scissors! As I discuss in the chapter "Body and Soul," I firmly believe in auras—the energy fields that surround a person and not only affect that person's health and mood, but also project his or her health and mood outward to the people around. If your hairstylist has the right aura, it will be in harmony with your own. If you and your hairstylist's auras do not jibe, you may wind up unhappy with your haircut, and you might even find that your hair does not grow as healthfully as it did before your unfortunate cut. There are people that I call cosmic vampires: they suck all the good energy out of you. So, never allow a stylist with negative energy near your hair. When people describe a stylist as having "una buena mano," or a good hand, it's because the stylist has good energy, and his or her cuts help your hair grow in healthy and strong—provided you do your part, of course. If this all sounds too New Agey and vague, following are some concrete things to help you match yourself with a great stylist.

A good stylist should be engaging and interested in what you have to say about your hair. Does the stylist have a hairstyle you like? Has he given other clients styles that you like? Does she spend time in consultation with you before cutting? Does she show you how much she's going to cut before wielding the scissors? The answer should to all of these questions should be yes.

Another important factor when selecting a stylist is to find someone who knows your hair type. This is where word of mouth and personal recommendations enter the equation. If you see someone on the street with a fabulous cut and a hair type similar to yours, ask her who cuts it. Trust me: she'll be nothing but flattered! My mother does it all the time! She'll stop a woman on the street and ask her where she gets her hair done. They chat, they exchange numbers. Needless to say, my mother always has glorious hair. In my case, I chose a stylist who understands that I like to experiment with new looks, and that my hair needs extra care and conditioning because of all the styling changes, climate changes, and stressors in my life.

A good hairstylist is part magician, part therapist, and part life coach. He or she should have an amazing talent for making your hair look its best, for listening to your tress tales of woe and worry, and for advising you if you are considering a dramatic change in color, texture, or length.

picking the right hairstyle

Your hair frames your face. You can use your hairstyle to accentuate your best features and play down the ones you're not wild about. Again, a good stylist should be able to advise you on which cuts will work best with your face. Here is some general advice about how different hairstyles work with different facial shapes.

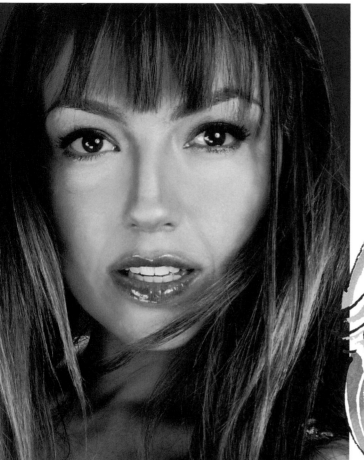

Bangs frame the eyes and layers emphasize the cheekbones

ROUND FACE

Create height and volume at the crown. Height and volume visually elongate the face.

Keep your hair at least at shoulder length, if possible. Cheek-baring lengths accentuate the roundness of the face.

Have layers cut along the sides, to narrow the face and create an illusion of more prominent cheekbones.

LONG FACE

Cut bangs wide and sharp, to visually "shorten" the face.

Keep the hair at chin length to add width to the lower portion of the face.

Avoid long, straight styles and one-length cuts, which draw attention to the length of the face.

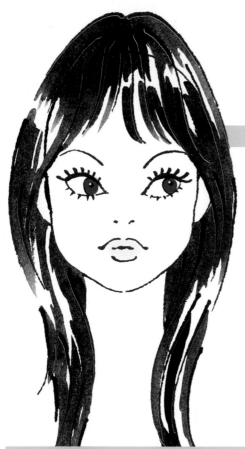

SQUARE FACE

Opt for longer styles with soft layers or curls, which can soften the angles of a square face.

Keep bangs lightweight and just long enough to hit along the top of the brows, a bit longer alongside the eyes.

Avoid sharp lines in a cut, or too-heavy bangs, because a too-blunt cut will accentuate your face's square shape.

HEART-SHAPED FACE

Create height around the crown.

Opt for width around the jawline; graduated layers visually even out the face.

Avoid a center part, which will draw the eye to the chin.

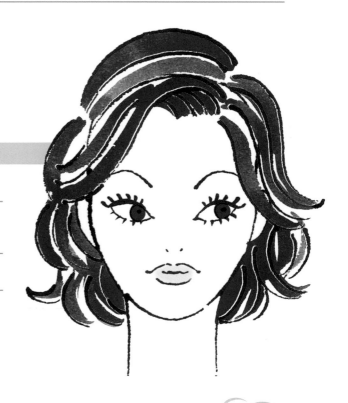

washing and conditioning

Because hair is my personal obsession, I can spend hours in the drugstore aisles, reading all the labels and picking through the different shampoos, conditioners, and styling products. When I'm stressed, I go to Ricky's or Sephora to see what the latest and greatest hair products are.

Picking the right shampoo and conditioner seems like it should be easy, but with all the different things we do to our hair, the choices can be complicated. You need to consider not only your hair and scalp type, but also the chemical processes you've put your hair through, the styling techniques you regularly use, and your environment. Since I've spent so much time staring at shelf after shelf of hair products and a lifetime trying them all out, here is a quick guide to help you make the choices easier.

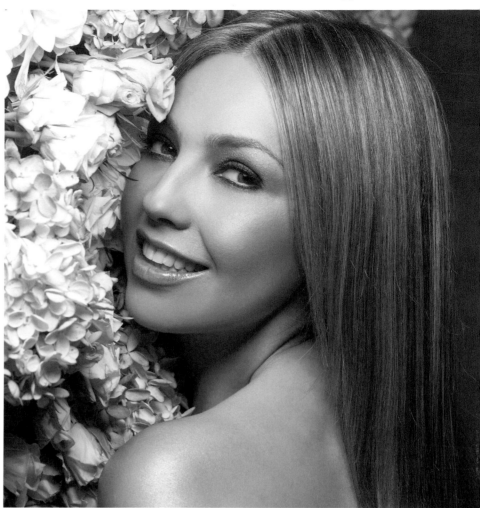

cleansing

IF YOU HAVE . . .	THEN CHOOSE . . .	IF YOU HAVE . . .	THEN CHOOSE . . .
Fine hair	Volumizing shampoo to boost your roots	Dry scalp	A cleanser that specifically targets this scalp condition
Curly hair	Hydrating shampoo, because curly hair tends to be drier than straight	Dandruff	Shampoo with pyrithione zinc or tea tree oil, to remove and prevent flakes
Oily hair	Clarifying shampoo to remove oily buildup and product residue	Relaxed or permed hair	Gentle, conditioning shampoo for processed hair
Dry hair	Moisturizing or hydrating shampoo	Color-treated hair	Shampoos for colored hair, which will clean without stripping or fading color

conditioner

IF YOU HAVE ...	THEN CHOOSE ...
Fine hair	A light daily conditioner that will not weigh the hair down
Curly hair	A rich moisturizing conditioner that will minimize frizz
Oily hair	A light conditioner applied only from the middle to the tips—not to the scalp
Dry hair	A moisturizing conditioner that is light enough that it won't weigh hair down

IF YOU HAVE ...	THEN CHOOSE ...
Dry scalp	A hydrating conditioner, but not too heavy if your hair is fine
Dandruff	A rich conditioner, because dandruff shampoo tends to be harsh on the hair
Relaxed or permed hair	Gentle, deep, or leave-in conditioner formulated specifically for processed hair
Color-treated hair	A rich leave-in conditioner with sunscreen to protect your color from the effects of the sun

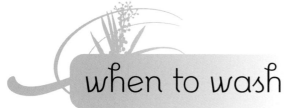

when to wash

How often you wash your hair is a personal choice, but few women actually need to wash their hair every single day. Overwashing strips your locks of their own natural oils, which protect your hair. How often you wash can also change with the seasons and the temperature. You might find that during hot weather, you will need to wash more often. You are the best judge of what needs to be done to your hair, and adapting your routine to respond to the season and your environment is the best way to keep your hair looking fabulous.

▩ CELEB SECRET REVEALED! ▩

Here is a beauty tip for a hot summer day, bien caliente: Before I go to the beach or for a dip in the pool, I wet my hair with tap water. I apply a deep-conditioning hair mask, pull my hair up into a ponytail, and let the sun "bake" it for a super-deep-conditioning treatment on the go. Doing this also will protect your hair: because it has already absorbed the water and the treatment, it won't be so affected by drying salt water or chlorine.

hair tlc

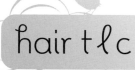

The more styling processes and treatments you subject your hair to, the more likely it will need care beyond the standard washing and conditioning. I have been on many a photo shoot where my hair has gone under the blow-dryer, the curling iron, the flat iron, and hot curlers—all in one day. Then I woke up the next morning and had to repeat the process. That's why deep-conditioning treatments are essential. A good deep-conditioning treatment repairs your hair and returns it to a healthy state—although it may take more than one treatment to get it there—and helps to minimize the damage that even normal heat styling will eventually have on your pelo.

If you've had chemical treatments such as color, hair relaxers, or perms, try a strengthening, protein-based conditioning treatment. These treatments help to restore the hair's elasticity and minimize breakage by strengthening the core of the hair and smoothing the outer cuticle, leaving you with luscious locks. When shopping for one, look for ingredients such as protein, panthenol, or fatty acids, or descriptors such as *strengthening* or *restructurizing*. To get the most out of the treatment, follow these steps:

Wash your hair with a clarifying shampoo to remove product buildup. Rinse well and squeeze out any excess water.

Apply a generous dollop of the conditioning treatment to your palms, rub it between your hands, and apply it to your hair, starting at the ends. (If your hair is fine, apply a smaller amount and avoid getting the product too near the scalp.)

Comb your hair with a wide-tooth comb to distribute the conditioner through to the ends.

Clip your hair on top of your head with a butterfly clip, and cover your head with a plastic shower cap.

Over the cap, cover your head with a warm towel, to allow the treatment to deeply penetrate your hair. Wait fifteen minutes.

Rinse well—and if you can stand it, do it with cold water. This closes the cuticles, sealing them down. Your hair should immediately look and feel smoother.

■ **HAIR EXPERIMENTS GONE AWRY** ■

When I launched myself as a solo artist, breaking off from my teen pop group, I wanted to introduce myself to the public with a whole new look. I thought that bleaching a lock of hair would be a cool idea. It would be like a signal to the world that I was stepping out! I put the worst thing in my hair to bleach it: facial hair bleach. I'm surprised I didn't end up with a bald spot, since facial hair bleach completely strips the hair. Later on, I thought if I tried Sun-in, it might give me sun-drenched highlights without the damage. I'd invite my girlfriends over, and we would drench our hair with Sun-in. Instead of a beautiful, buttery chunk of blonde, I got orangey-yellow hair. It was so damaging to my hair that my split ends practically traveled all the way up to my roots. It took me at least three or four years to regrow healthy hair to the length I am used to wearing it.

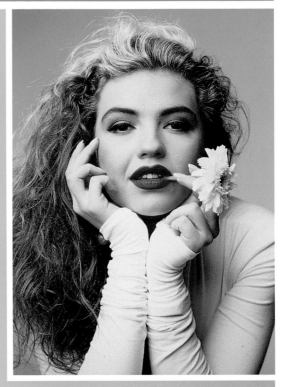

Since then, I've experimented in more moderation. You can play with your look without going to extremes. I have gone from dark brunette (on some of my soap operas) to reddish auburn to a light brunette with caramel highlights. The lesson here: If you really want to bleach your hair, leave it to the experts.

styling products 101

Styling products are like makeup for the hair: choose the right formulas, and you will look estupenda. Choose the wrong ones, and your hair will look frumpy. The "right" products are determined by a combination of the look you are hoping to achieve and your own experimentation. Consult your hairdresser on what he or she uses to achieve your dashing 'do, or give yourself time to read the labels on the hair products at the drugstore or beauty store.

GEL This basic styling tool serves so many functions, from giving a high hold to protecting your hair from heat styling to keeping curls from frizzing if you air-dry your hair. Mixing gel with styling cream, straightening balm, or serum boosts the hold factor of the other products.

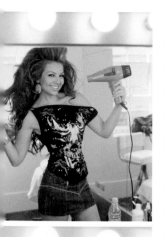

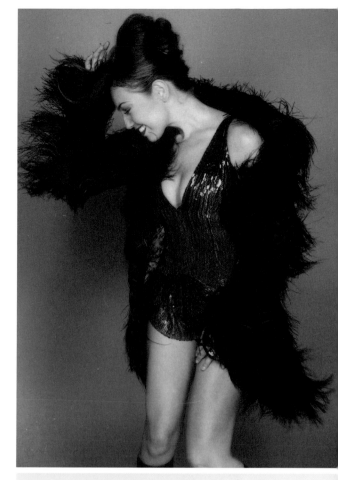

MOUSSE You may be tempted to dismiss mousse as a throwback to the '80s, but this product is great at giving a frothy volume boost to short hairstyles or to big, telenovela–Miss Universe styles. It also works well with fine hair. Apply when hair is wet before blow-drying or to dry when you want to pump up your style.

POMADE A waxy product, pomade works wonders on dry hair to create a piece-y smooth look. Use it after you've blow-dried your hair to smooth wiry flyaways and tame your ends. Pomade is also great to groom the fuzzy baby hairs around the hairline.

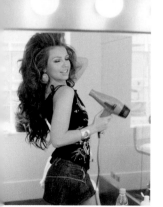

SERUM Shine serums are silicone-based liquids that, when applied to curly or straight hair, eliminate frizz and give hair a high shine. To keep hair glossy—not greasy— avoid using too much! Because serum coats the hair so effectively, if you use it regularly, wash with a clarifying shampoo once or twice a month to remove buildup.

it took more than bobby pins to get hair this high...

STRAIGHTENING BALM A good straightening balm serves a number of functions: it protects your hair from heat styling, relaxes hair's natural curl or wave, prevents frizzing, and helps keep hair straight until the next shampoo. Apply it to wet hair before you heat style.

STYLING CREAM A must-have for women who color, straighten, or curl their hair, styling cream protects the hair from heat, moisturizes the hair, and leaves it soft and silky. It is especially good for curly hair because it hydrates as it helps to style.

■ **CELEB SECRET REVEALED!** ■

Every time I go to the beach, I order a dozen clear beers (i.e., not lager or ale). No, I don't drink them; I pour them on my hair and allow the sun to dry my hair with the beer in it, because the bran in the beer brings out beautiful highlights. I smell like a drunk for a little while, but it works!

VOLUMIZER The most effective volumizers, or thickeners, are sprays applied to the roots to boost body before you style your hair. Volumizers are spot styling treatments, meant to be applied where you need the volume, such as at the roots or at the crown, as opposed to the entire hair shaft.

HEAT PROTECTANT Heat protectants come in many forms: gels, sprays, balms. Sometimes straightening balms have heat-protectant properties in the formula. Whichever formula you choose, the key is to try to incorporate it into your hair-care regimen if you heat-style your hair regularly—especially if you use flat irons.

HAIR SPRAY A fave of the telenovela and beauty-queen set, hair spray is the last step in a styling regimen. I was an Aqua Net devotee in the '80s. My hair defied gravity. Used sparingly, hair spray is excellent at holding a style and keeping it fresh throughout the day. It should be used only on dried, styled hair.

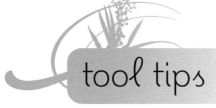

tool tips

Hairstyling tools are the makeup brushes and eyelash curlers for your tresses. It makes sense to invest wisely in these items, so you will get the effect you are trying to achieve and will have lasting tools that won't break every time they accidentally drop on your bathroom floor.

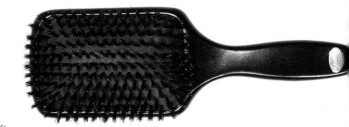

FLAT BRUSHES These brushes have an oval or rectangular back and bristles set in a slight curve. They are used for smoothing the hair and for brushing out tangles and hairstyles. Boar bristles, or a mix of boar and synthetic bristles, are excellent for smoothing the hair and redistributing oil from the roots to the length of the hair shaft.

ROUND BRUSHES Wide, round brushes are best for straightening and smoothing hair in conjunction with a blow-dryer. They give you the tight grip you need on your hair, to hold it taut while you are drying it.

RAT-TAILED COMB This fine-tooth comb is excellent for back combing the hair to create volume. Use its long tail to create parts.

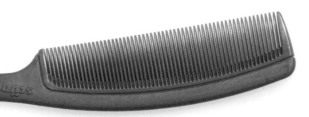

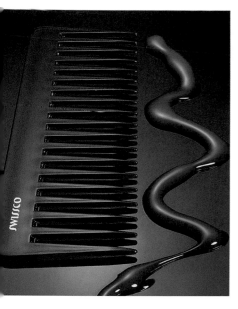

WIDE-TOOTH COMB This type of comb works best on wet hair to detangle it. Hair is weakest when it's wet, and this forgiving comb won't tear at your tangles. A wide-tooth comb also will distribute conditioning treatments evenly throughout the hair.

CERAMIC CURLING IRON The more settings you have, the better you will be able to place a curling iron on the lowest setting that will give you the style you want. Different curling irons with different barrel widths create a wide variety of looks. Check out the sexy, tousled 'do you can create with a large-barrel curling iron (see page 92) and the tightly curled, face-framing 'do you can get with a small-barrel curling iron (see page 93).

HOT ROLLERS High-quality hot rollers should have a velvetlike rod to really grip and smooth the ends. They also should heat evenly and not burn your fingers if you touch them in the right places. Hot rollers are held in place with pins or with clamps, which come included in the hot roller set. I prefer the clamps—they are easier to work with.

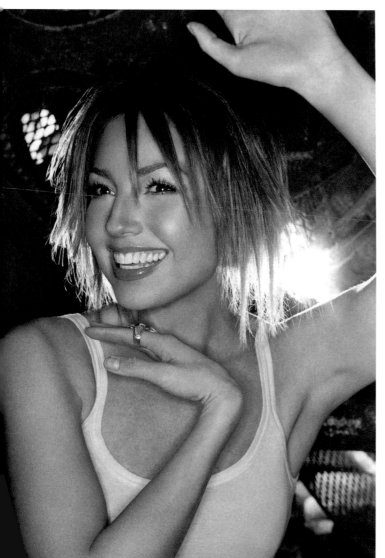

HIGH-WATTAGE IONIC BLOW-DRYER You need at least eighteen hundred watts for serious styling. Select a dryer with independent heat and speed settings, so you can use a high speed at a low heat. It also should have a cool-blast button, which helps to smooth the hair cuticles. Ionic dryers are a relatively new development. Without getting into the science of positively and negatively charged ions, I'll just say that these dryers help seal the hair cuticle, which protects it from heat damage and ensures a high shine to the hair. You also need to make sure the dryer has a straightening attachment, which directs the heat and air into a concentrated area, making styling easier.

FLAT IRON Look for one with ceramic plates, which distribute the heat evenly. As with a curling iron, look for one with several heat options, so you can use the lowest heat necessary to straighten your hair.

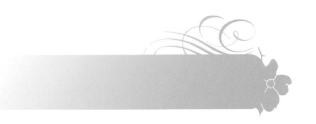

hair makeovers

Now that we have the basic products and tools down, I want to show you how to make the best of the hair you have when you wake up in the morning (so you don't always have to default to a ponytail!), and how to style it differently for a completely new look. We took four models with different hair types that match the broad range of hair textures common to Latinas and gave each of them two looks.

straight hair

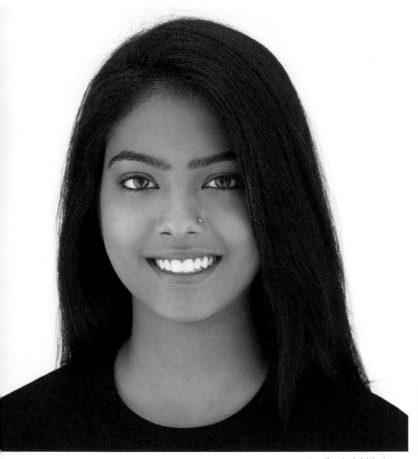

naturally straight hair

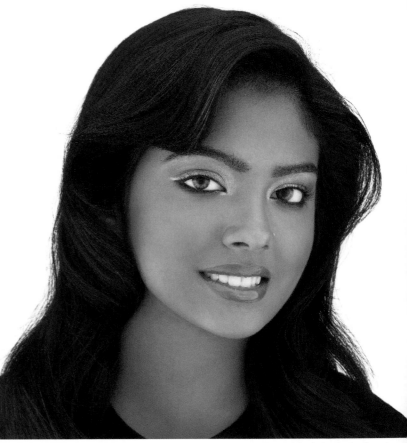

naturally straight hair—hot rollered

Long, straight hair is the closest thing to wash-and-go hair. The key to keeping it glossy and healthy is a good diet and regular trims. You can either air-dry or blow-dry straight hair, though drying with a blow-dryer with your head upside down will give an extra boost of body to your roots. Once the hair is dried, all you need to style long, straight hair is a dab of a light stying cream on the ends (if they're prone to dryness), followed by a few drops of shine serum. With both products, squeeze or pump a small amount onto your palms. Rub your hands together and apply it with your hands over the surface of the hair. Through the day, if your ends tend to get straggly or fly away, a quick, light application of pomade or gel will tame strays. Use these products lightly—too much will leave the hair looking damp and lifeless.

To change your look, use hot rollers to give super-straight tresses the wavy, sexy style of an old-school screen siren. Women with other hair textures can also benefit from hot rollers; in the first step below, simply apply a straightening balm to damp hair, instead of volumizing mousse or spray.

❋ Apply volumizing mousse or spray to fine, damp hair, especially at the roots.

❋ Allow your hair to completely dry.

❋ Apply shine serum from the middle of your hair to the ends. Avoid your roots, because shine products tend to weigh hair down and the goal here is lush, weightless volume.

❋ If you want tighter curls that have longer hold, apply hair spray instead.

❋ Using a fine-tooth comb, divide your hair into three parts, as if you were creating a mohawk with a two-inch-wide swath of hair running from your hairline to the nape of your neck. Secure the two side sections with clips.

❋ Starting at the front of the middle section, use a comb to separate a smaller section of hair at the forehead and comb it forward.

❋ Pull this section of hair taut and place a heated roller one to two inches from the end. Be careful not to burn your fingers.

❋ Tuck the ends of the roller under the taut hair and slowly roll the curler back toward your forehead. Secure with a pin or a clamp.

❋ With the fine-tooth comb, separate another small section of hair directly behind the first, and repeat the process with this section. Depending on the length and thickness of your hair, and on the width of the hot roller barrels themselves, you should end up with ten to fifteen rolled sections.

❋ Roll the sections on the sides of the head downward.

❋ Wait fifteen to twenty minutes for the rollers to completely cool, then remove them, starting with the first roller at the forehead.

❋ Loosen the curls by brushing them with a flat brush. Flip your head over and brush the underside of your hair, to keep its volume.

curly hair

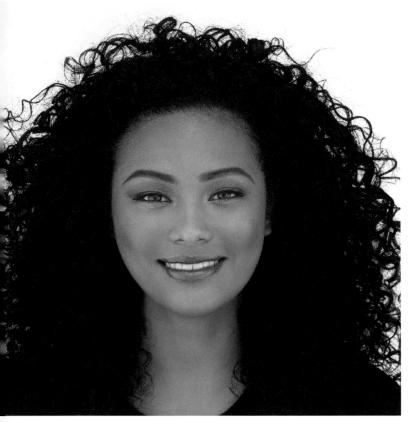

naturally curly hair

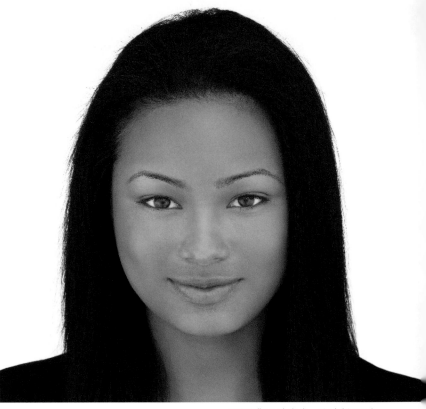

naturally curly hair—straightened

Tight corkscrew curls can also be wash-and-go. The trick is to keep the curl while avoiding the frizz. To do this, keep hairbrushes away from damp, newly washed hair. Instead, groom with a wide-tooth comb. Always use a leave-in conditioner, because curly hair is prone to drying and breaking. Follow with a mix of gel to hold the curl and a few drops of serum to avoid frizz. When you can, give your hair a break from the blow-dryer and let it dry naturally. When the weather or time does not permit air-drying, use a diffuser attachment on your blow-dryer, to disperse the air as it dries your hair. When using a diffuser, it is critical to cup the curls rather than scrunch them, which will almost always result in frizz.

To make even tighter, higher curls, as we did here, start with your naturally curly dry hair. Dampen dry hair with water and a quick spritz of hair spray. Scrunch the curls by the fistful, holding each bunch for about thirty seconds, until the hair spray has had a chance to hold. You can also use butterfly clips: spritz your dry hair with hair spray, scrunch your hair into a bunch, and use a butterfly clip to hold the bunch in place until it dries completely.

Curly girls can go silky straight with the help of the right tools and technique. With a blow-dryer and a round brush, try the following method.

✳ Start with freshly washed and conditioned hair. Apply a heat-protective styling balm.

✳ Towel your hair dry and squeeze out excess water.

✻ Blast the roots with a blow-dryer at high speed and high heat. Lift your hair at the roots with your fingers to dry it section by section, to get out the wetness. Dry the rest of your hair until it is damp and no longer dripping.

✻ Make a part across your head from ear to ear. Clip the front section aside.

✻ Place the straightening attachment on the nozzle of the blow-dryer. Divide the back hair into smaller sections. If it makes it easier, separate the section you will be working on, and clip the rest of the wet hair so it does not get in the way. With hair this curly, you have to dry it section by section.

✻ Turn the dryer on high heat at a high-speed setting. Use a round brush to dry each back section, concentrating on drying the roots completely and smoothing and drying the ends until they are dry to the touch. Use the brush to grip each section, starting at the roots. Hold the hair taut as you pull the brush down to the ends. Once the back section is completely dry, release the front section.

✻ Separate the front section into three smaller sections. Dry and smooth each section separately and completely.

✻ Once your entire head is dry, warm a smoothing serum between your palms and apply it from mid-shaft to the ends of your freshly styled hair.

What if you want hair as perfectly pin-straight as your hairstylist can make it? Achieving the look with a blow-dryer alone is truly an art. If it doesn't give you the satisfaction you're seeking, try using a flat iron. Flat irons are wildly popular with Latinas, because they create straight hair that won't frizz or curl even in Miami-type humidity. But if they are used improperly, flat irons can seriously damage your hair, because they require such intense heat. The trick is to move the heated iron from the roots to the ends of your hair in a steady, fluid motion. If you want to try your hand at using a flat iron, give the following steps a go.

✻ Use a flat iron only on completely dry hair. If your hair is still wet, you're basically boiling it! If you have ultra-curly hair like our models, you will have to blow-dry your hair straight. If your hair is wavy, you can dry it normally and use the iron on wavy, dry hair.

✻ Divide your hair into sections.

✻ Apply a heat-protective styling spray to each section before placing the section between the plates. Run the heated iron from the roots to the ends of the section. You should have to do this only once or twice per section if you are working with a high-quality straightening iron.

✻ Repeat with each remaining section.

✻ When you have straightened each section to your satisfaction, apply a few drops of shine serum to your palm. Rub it between your palms and gently run the palms over your hair, concentrating on the ends.

wavy hair

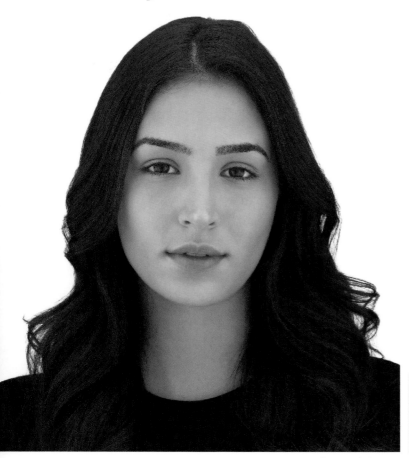

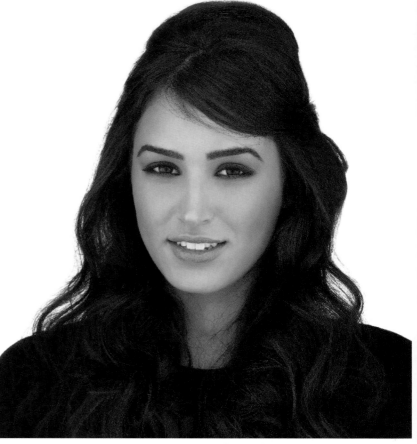

naturally wavy hair

naturally wavy hair—in a sex kitten style

Naturally wavy hair is totally sexy. To get it to look its glorious best, the goal should be to prevent frizz. Keep it as healthy as possible and use pomade or gel on the ends to prevent frizzing. Air-dry your hair if weather and time permit, or use a blow-dryer with a diffuser attachment. Serum can be effective at keeping away frizz, but use it lightly, because the beauty of wavy hair is in its body, and too much serum can flatten the natural lift of the hair.

Wavy girls can easily get sex kitten hair. This look re-creates a sexy Brigitte Bardot–type hairstyle from the '60s. You achieve the height by back-combing the crown. Create the loose spirals at the sides and back with a wide-barrel curling iron.

❋ Section off a three-inch-wide swath of hair starting from the front and going back toward the crown.

❋ Use a rat-tailed comb to tease the hair in this section, starting at the crown. Hold the section upward with one hand, place the comb three inches above the roots, and comb downward toward the scalp. Repeat vigorously, working toward the front hairline. The hair should almost be standing upright on its own.

❋ Use a brush to smooth the front area of the section you have just teased, starting from the hairline and brushing backward toward the crown. Brush lightly, because you don't want to undo all the height you have achieved by teasing. The volume created by the teasing underneath will create a cushion of height. Smooth the top layer toward the back and secure it with a clip or bobby pins.

❉ Apply gel or styling cream to the loose sides and ends of the hair.

❉ Separate hair into two- to three-inch sections on the sides and back. Grasp the end of a section with a wide-barrel curling iron. Roll the section around the barrel of the iron and hold the hair in place for a few seconds. Repeat the process on each section throughout the sides and back of the head.

❉ After the sections have been curled, rub a small amount of styling cream between your palms and gently separate and pull the curls to create a softer, looser, less "done" appearance.

relaxed hair

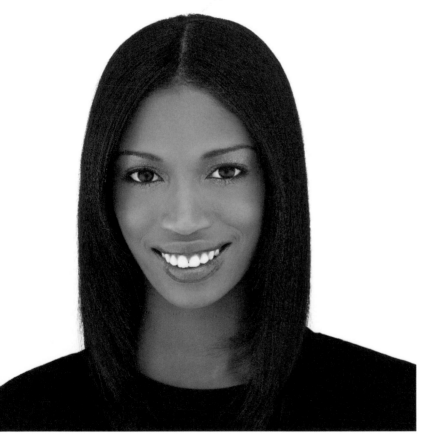

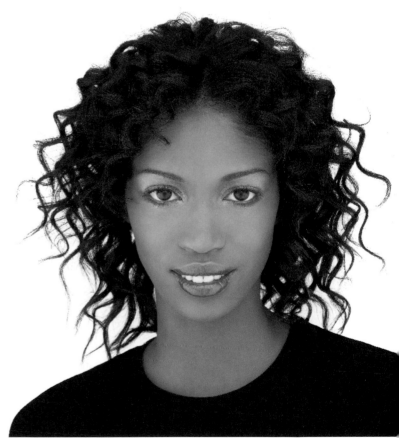

relaxed hair

relaxed hair—with curls

Relaxed hair still needs to be blown dry to achieve a smooth, straight look. Because relaxed hair no longer has tight curls, you can smooth it with a quick, time-saving blow-dry. Take care to keep the hair dryer moving, so the heat does not scorch the processed hair.

❉ Start with freshly washed and conditioned hair. Apply a heat-protective styling balm.

❋ Blast the roots with the blow-dryer at high speed. Lift your hair at the roots with your fingers to dry it section by section. Your roots should be completely dry, while the ends remain damp. Pay close attention to the crown and back of your head. Get the roots in these areas as dry as possible.

❋ Make a part across the crown of your head from ear to ear. Clip the front section aside.

❋ Place the straightening attachment on the nozzle of your blow-dryer. Divide the back hair into smaller sections.

❋ With the blow-dryer set on high heat at a high-speed setting, use a round brush to dry each section, concentrating on drying the roots completely and smoothing and drying the ends until they are dry to the touch. Use the brush to grip each section starting at the roots. Hold the hair taut as you pull the brush down to the ends.

❋ Separate the front section into three smaller sections. Dry and smooth each section separately and completely.

❋ Once your entire head is dry, rub a smoothing serum between your palms and apply it from mid-shaft to the ends of your freshly styled hair.

A small-barrel curling iron is a great tool for getting tight spiral curls. The trick is to work quickly, so as not to overheat the ends.

❋ Begin with dry hair. Ideally, you have blow-dried the hair straight so that your ends are nice and smooth. This will ensure that the curl takes better.

❋ Apply a heat-protective gel or styling cream to dry hair.

❋ Using a rat-tailed comb, separate a small, one-inch section of hair.

❋ Grasp this section of hair with the curling iron as near to the roots as possible. Pull the iron to the end and wind the hair around the barrel in a spiral formation. Hold the hair in the curling iron for a few seconds, just long enough for the curl to take hold.

❋ Release the hair, gently unwinding the strand from the barrel. The curl should stay in formation.

❋ Repeat the process, working around the head section by section. Take special care with the curls that frame the face.

❋ Once all the curls have been set and cooled, use your fingers to gently take each individual curl and separate it into two.

❋ With the curls that fall around the face, pull the separated curls down and toward the face. The final effect should be a frame of curls that surround the face.

home remedies

One of my favorite remedios caseros is an avocado deep-conditioning hair mask. Unlike other treatments that require you to wash your hair, apply the treatment, wait fifteen to thirty minutes, then get back in the shower and rinse the treatment out, you apply this one before you wash your hair. This hydrating mask is great for very dry hair that has been exposed to blow-drying or curling irons. If you have seriously damaged hair, you may need to apply a deep conditioner like this twice a week. If your hair is normal to oily, try it once a month.

✳ Scrape out half a ripe, soft avocado. Mash it up in a bowl to make a paste. For extra moisturizing help, mix in some olive oil. You have to eyeball the amount of oil based on how dry your hair is. Don't add too much oil or you will lose the paste-type texture making the mixture harder to work with.

✳ Dampen your hair with water.

✳ Apply the avocado paste to your hair, concentrating on the ends. Use a wide-tooth comb to ensure that the paste is distributed evenly throughout your hair.

✳ Cover your hair with a plastic shower cap and leave the paste in for thirty minutes.

✳ Rinse the paste out, then wash and condition your hair as usual.

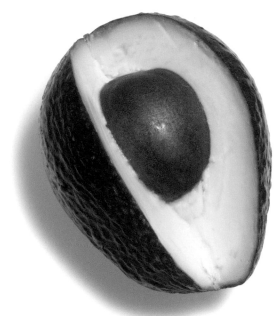

My second, super-easy hair mask recipe: a jar of mayonnaise. Apply an entire small jar to dry hair. Make sure to saturate your hair completely from ends to roots. Clip your hair up and put a plastic shower cap on your head. Leave the mayo on for thirty to forty minutes, then take a shower and wash your hair as normal. You will smell like a salad, but your hair will be glorious!

█ CELEB SECRET REVEALED! █

Keep a jar of cooled chamomile tea at hand when you take a shower. After you have washed and conditioned your hair, pour the cooled tea over your mane. Don't rinse it out. The chamomile brings out the varied highlights in your hair and leaves a brilliant sheen.

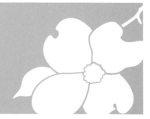

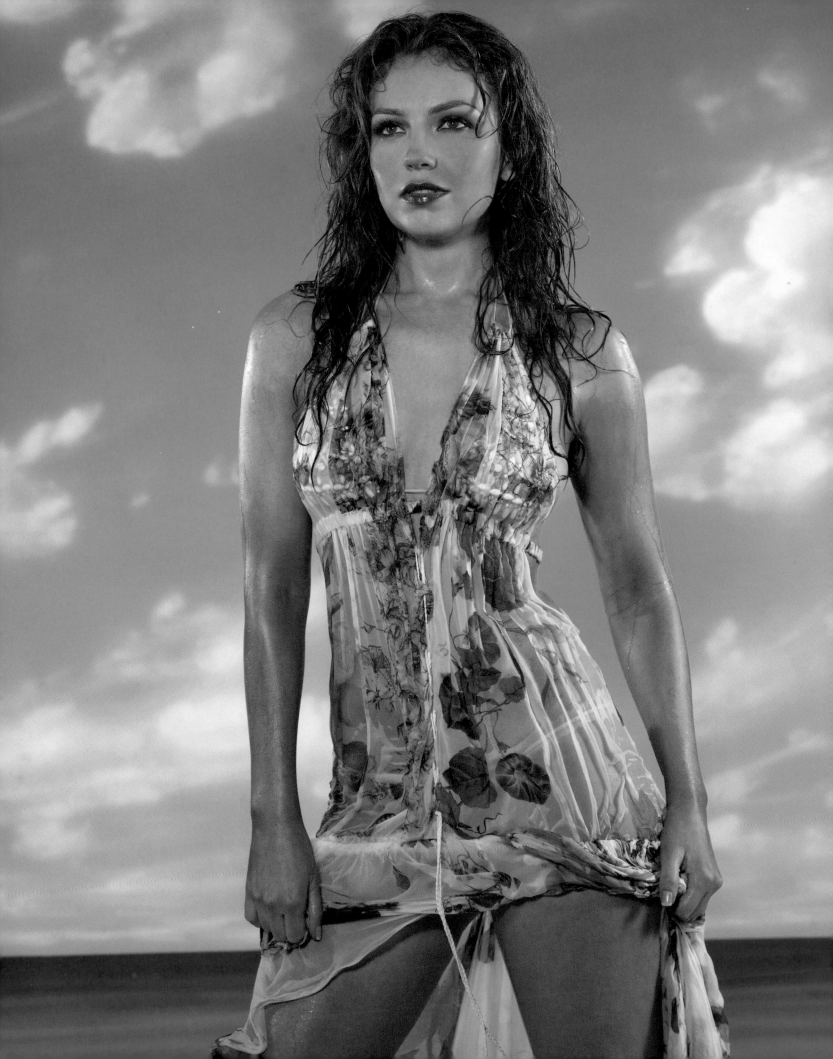

smooth and polished

BODY, HANDS, AND FEET

Skin care for the body is just as important as skin care for the face. I learned this lesson the hard way. Years ago, I was in Cuernavaca, a resort town in south-central Mexico, to do a concert. I brought a girlfriend with me, and we sat beside the hotel pool and suntanned. We ordered lobster for lunch, which came with a side of cold whipped butter. We decided to slather ourselves in the butter, which we thought would soften our skin and give it a beautiful, brown look. Instead, we basted under the bright, hot sun. The lobster we ate was slightly less red than we were at the end of that little experiment. That night at my performance, I am positive that the people in the first four rows thought I looked like one of the characters from the Fantastic Four—and not the sexy blonde chick, either. I had to sing and dance, when all I really wanted was to be dipped in a vat of aloe vera gel and take aspirin for the pain.

I now know that there are better ways to pamper yourself and love the skin you're in. I'll show you how.

exfoliating

For your body, exfoliation is the way to sexy, smooth skin. Exfoliation removes dry, scaly, ashen skin from the surface and polishes your piel to a buffed sheen. Exfoliators have all sorts of beneficial ingredients to bring out the best in your skin, from sugar, which swipes away the old cells, to caffeine, which helps minimize the appearance of cellulite. I use salt- or sugar-based scrubs mixed

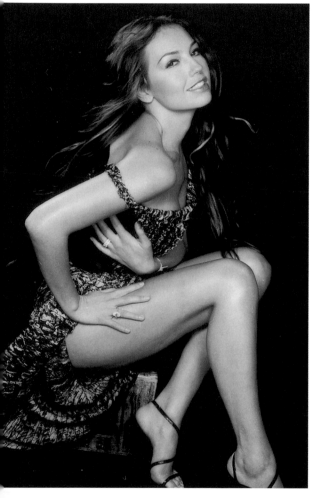

with natural oils, which leave my skin feeling absolutely heavenly. The best scrubs have a nice balance of abrasive ingredients and rich oils or creams: they don't leave the skin feeling greasy, and they rub just enough to leave even tricky areas that need more scrubbing—such as the elbows, knees, and ankles—smooth to the touch. My favorite exfoliator is the mango scrub by Carol's Daughter.

Instead of looking at exfoliation as a chore, I view it as a pampering treatment. I do it in the shower, starting with my feet and working my way up, giving an extra scrub to ankles, knees, and elbows. There are other ways to exfoliate besides using an abrasive scrub, including using a loofah sponge and a special scrubby towel for hard-to-reach areas such as your back. But if giving yourself a vigorous scrub-down rubs you the wrong way, you can get exfoliating action with body creams that have alpha hydroxy acids in the formula. AHAs will do the work for you by sloughing off the dead skin cells and leaving you with gleaming fresh skin. I exfoliate more in the summer, but still do it at least once a week in the winter to keep my skin glowing.

CELEB SECRET REVEALED!

Next time you are lounging on the beach, use wet sand to exfoliate your skin, particularly around the ankles, heels, soles of your feet, knees, and elbows. My sister Titi likes to say, "Te quita la ciudad de encima"—it sloughs the city off your skin. It's easy, and it's free. You might even want to make like a sexy diva and ask your sweetie to do it for you. Then, after you wash the sand away, up the sexiness factor even more by having your honey apply sunscreen to your newly softened legs and feet.

moisturizing

I am a little moody when it comes to moisturizing my body:
I like to do what feels right at the moment. Sometimes I apply baby
oil when I'm still wet in the shower, then towel off. If I'm in a more
luxurious, pampering state of mind, I break out the rich, expensive
creams. Sometimes I do a light body mist, using one with oil and
maybe a light fragrance. In this step of your body-care routine,
you can be spontaneous and self-expressive. The ultimate goal is
to take care of your skin and, especially if you are preparing to
apply self-tanner, keep it supple and soft. Don't forget to rub the
oil, cream, or mist on your ankles and feet. They need it too!

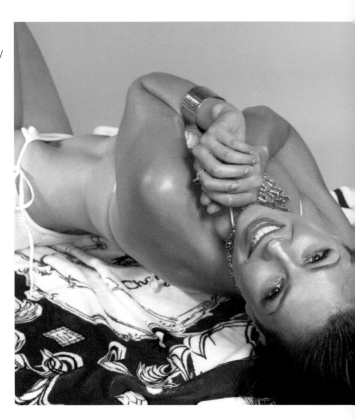

Besides how I'm feeling, I also take into account the weather.
During the winter months, I practically bathe myself in rich
creams. In the summer I stick to lighter formulas that will still
leave my skin with a smooth gleam. For my hands I use a
moisturizer with sunscreen in the formula year-round.

self-tanning

There's nothing sexier than beautiful piel morena, so who can blame us for wanting to pump up the tan when
summer comes? Most women are drawn to the glow that the sun gives, but there are better ways to get that
radiance than basting in butter, like I did. Use a self-tanner. There are so many good ones on the market today
that can give you a healthy-looking glow. Today you can find self-tanners in several different hues. But be careful.
A botched self-tanner application means a week of heavy-duty exfoliation and full-coverage clothing.

Also keep in mind that not all self-tanners are created equal. I hate self-tanners that *smell* like self-tanners.
Light gel formulas have the least offensive smell, but I prefer sprays. Besides easily getting into all those nooks
and crannies—between your toes, in your navel—sprays leave behind little odor.

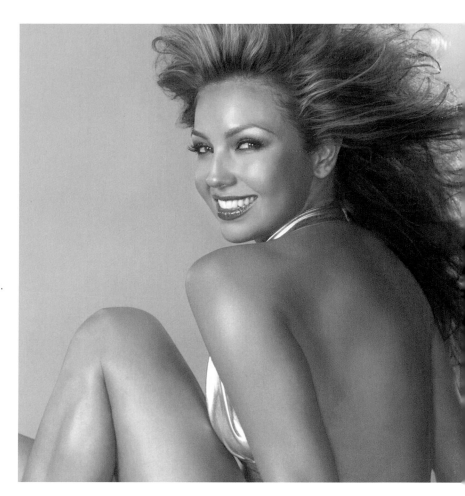

If you feel slightly intimidated by the thought of applying a tanner yourself, you may wonder if spray-tanning booths might not be an easier option. I've never used these booths. I feel like the spray might get into my lungs and turn them orange. I'd rather just grab a can of spray-on self-tanner and do it myself, in my bathroom. It's really not that difficult. Here are my step-by-step instructions on how to give yourself a fantastic tan.

❋ Begin with freshly shaved legs. If you wax, wait at least twenty-four hours before you start the self-tanning process.

❋ Use a scrub with tiny beads to fully exfoliate your skin. Pay extra attention to the rough areas around the knees, elbows, ankles, and feet, because they will soak up any extra self-tanner.

❋ Use a moisturizer to create a barrier cream on areas that do not get tanned when you suntan naturally. This prevents your tan-from-a-can from screaming "fake" every time you wave at someone and she sees that the palm of your hand has become orange and streaky. Be sure to apply the moisturizer between your fingers and toes, on and under the nails, on your elbows, and in your belly button. It's important to shave, exfoliate, and moisturize before you use self-tanner, because the tanner blends more easily, and you are less likely to get telltale marks around your knees and ankles.

❋ Stand in the bathtub and hold the can six to eight inches away from your skin. Spray on the self-tanner beginning from the toes and moving upward in small circles. Hold the spray can farther away (eight or so inches) when spraying your feet, knees, and elbows.

❋ Think about yoga moves when spraying your back: raise one arm, bend it at the elbow, and point the nozzle down over your shoulder to reach your upper back. For your lower back, use your other arm to reach behind your waist and spray upward.

❋ Be sure to spray the neck, the sides of the body, and under your boobies: all of these areas are commonly missed when you're self-tanning.

❋ Wash your hands immediately after you are finished. Scrub your fingers with a nail brush.

❋ Wait at least twenty to thirty minutes before putting on clothes, going to bed, or applying moisturizer. You have no other choice but to stand there naked.

❋ Be generous with the body lotion after the self-tanner has fully dried. Self-tanner tends to dry the skin; applying extra lotion or cream after the formula has dried helps the faux tan last longer and keeps the dryness to a minimum. Self-tanner should last three to five days.

❋ Goofed? Dark spots—places where you didn't blend well or where you applied too much—are hard to cover up. Your best bet is to use the new skin lotions with reflective shimmer particles in the formula, which will minimize the appearance of such mistakes. A light spot is slightly easier to correct: use a Q-tip to spot-apply some self tanner.

❋ The new body lotions with diluted self-tanner in the formula are pretty mistake-proof. The color builds with each daily application, so you are not trying to leap ahead three shades darker in one application. Just apply it daily like you do your regular moisturizing lotion. For a DIY approach, mix your regular self-tanner with your regular moisturizing body lotion. It will have the same effect.

self-tanning on the face

I personally do not use self-tanner on my face, but a lot of muchachas really love the subtle glow that self-tanner creates. Some hints for proper application:

❋ Start with a clean, exfoliated face.

❋ Mix a little facial self-tanner with your moisturizer; this ensures you do not go too dark too fast.

❋ Apply first to the cheeks and forehead, and blend to the rest of the areas of your face from there.

❋ Take special care around brows and the hairline, where the self-tanner can clump and become a dark, splotchy mess. To avoid patches, apply sparingly in these areas and blend very, very well.

❋ Don't forget your neck, or you will get a chinstrap that won't come off with makeup remover. Blend, carajo, blend!

CELEB SECRET REVEALED!

There's nothing worse than an obviously fake tan. You know—that awful orange hue. I've seen too many actresses on the red carpet looking like they'd rolled around in Cheetos dust before putting on their couture gown. That is why, for a big event, I prefer using body makeup instead of self-tanner. I apply it sparingly. I like my skin color and my skin tone. Body makeup doesn't change my skin tone, but enhances it.

areas that need tlc

We all know how important it is to use a sunscreen on the face every day. But what about the décolletage? The bust, the chest, and the neck are three of the most ignored areas when it comes to a woman's skin-care regimen. Here are my must-dos:

❋ Use sunscreen on these areas daily—apply the same one you use on your face or buy special hand cream with an SPF in the formula.

❋ Invest in a tightening, toning bust cream. Will it do the work of a plastic surgeon or a Wonderbra? No, but it can't hurt, and you'll find that with regular use, the delicate skin in these areas will take on a smoother, more even-toned appearance.

❋ Include the neck when removing your makeup at night, and even your cleavage, if you have been so bold as to use bronzer or highlighter to amplify your curvas.

❋ Use upward strokes when applying cream to your neck, going from the base of the neck toward the chin. Better yet, use the index and middle fingers to gently "tap" upward in a gentle circular motion. Facialists say that this stimulates the skin and keeps it tight. Has science proved that it works? I don't know, but it feels great.

cellulite creams: do they work?

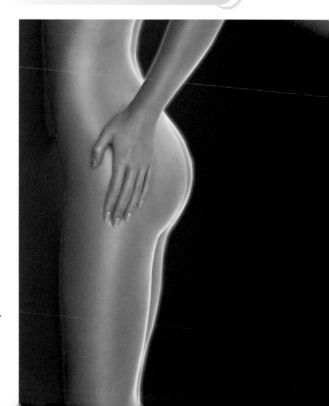

Like most women, I believe that cellulite is my sworn enemy. If there existed a cream or laser or magic potion that would blast that orange-peel-looking junk out of my body, I'd be the first in line to try it. Cellulite is so evil that even las flacas have it! The newest crop of cellulite creams help to minimize the appearance of cellulite mostly by virtue of the caffeine in their formulas. Because caffeine is a diuretic, it eliminates excess water or bloat from these areas of the skin, making the cellulite less noticeable. These creams won't leave you with the taut, unrippled skin of a six-year-old, but they can help you feel better about your body.

The other weapon to wield against cellulite is self-tanner. Because it darkens the skin, it can help to camouflage the wrinkly surface a little bit.

SKIN-CARE BUZZWORDS

This is the celebrity super-secret beauty cure for cellulite: Preparation H and Epsom salts. This little beauty trick will suck up all the excess puffiness right out of the treated area, minimizing the appearance of cellulite—at least for the time it takes to have a fun beach party! Consult with your doctor or dermatologist before trying this treatment as some people may have an allergic skin reaction to Epsom Salts and Preparation H. You will need:

✳ Bandage wraps (the kind you get at the drugstore if you have sprained something; you will need enough to cover your thighs and butt)

✳ Epsom salt

✳ Two tubes of Preparation H

✳ Saran Wrap

Soak the bandages in a solution of warm water and Epsom salts. Pour the entire box of Epsom salt into a 3-quart bowl to make a concentrated mixture.

While the bandages are soaking, apply Preparation H directly to your skin over the areas that have cellulite. Cover the area completely with the cream and allow it to absorb into the skin.

Wring out the bandages so they are damp with the solution, but not dripping.

Wrap your thighs in the bandages.

Over the bandages, wrap Saran Wrap around your thighs and butt. This will prevent dripping.

Keep the wraps on for twenty to thirty minutes.

mano a mano

I can't stand unkempt fingernails. I'll go with bare nails before letting my uñas get chipped and scraggly looking. When I see someone with picked-at or bitten nails, I immediately think that perhaps they are troubled people, insecure or histéricos.

Nail styles come and go. As an actress, I have had every type of nail length, design, and treatment imaginable. I have had dragon-lady acrylics and French manicures and short tips buffed to a high sheen, but my favorite nail look remains the same: short, with a sheer, creamy nail polish. This is also the easiest look to create and maintain yourself—no manicurist required.

My Sunday mani-pedi ritual is sacrosanct. I do it every week, without fail. My manicure lasts a full week because I do it

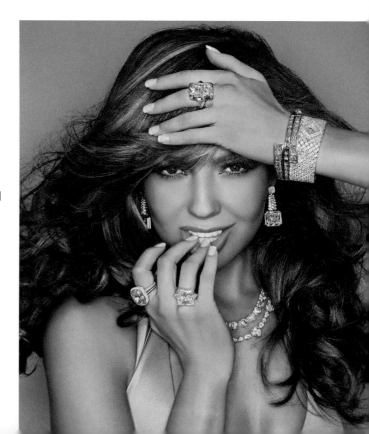

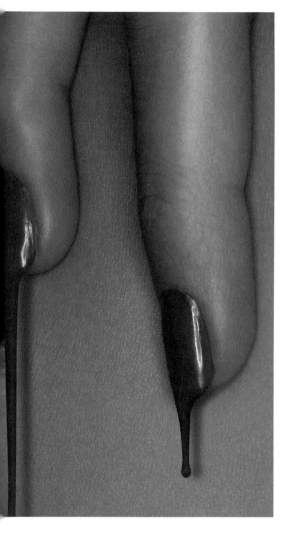

regularly and I use my secret super-fast top coat, Seche, to keep my nails from chipping. Here is my no-fail home manicure method:

❋ Remove nail polish with a gentle, nonacetone remover that won't dry your nails.

❋ Trim your nails using nail scissors, keeping a consistent length. Nine long nails and one short one just looks wrong. Keep them all the same length!

❋ File the tips gently with a fine-grain emery board. File in one direction, which will make your nails less likely to peel. I favor a square look, but it's fun to experiment with oval and pointed shapes.

❋ If you have ridges on your nails, use a buffer to even the surface.

❋ Apply cuticle balm, a thick, rich-textured cream that you rub into the nails and cuticles. Soak your fingertips in warm water for no longer than three to four minutes.

❋ Dry your hands, then gently push back your cuticles using a metal cuticle pusher with some cotton wrapped around the end. Wooden cuticle pushers can carry bacteria. Since you change the cotton with each use, there is no danger of that with a metal cuticle pusher.

❋ Use nail polish remover to wipe any excess balm or moisture off the nails.

❋ Apply a base coat, preferably a strengthening one, to make your nails more resilient. Try to avoid applying color to the nail directly, because repeatedly using color directly on the naked nail can lead to discoloration, giving your nails an icky yellowish appearance. Extend the base coat along edges of the tips and, if length allows, underneath the edge of the nail. Wait at least two minutes before applying color.

❋ Apply the polish, with the first stroke going down the center of the nail from base to tip and the second and third stroke on either side. Wait at least two minutes, to allow some of the color to harden. It seems like an eternity when you are polishing your own nails, but it is worth the wait. Consider it a mini-meditation session to calm the mind.

❋ Apply a second coat, following the same stroke pattern as the first.

❋ Wait two minutes and apply a fast drier. I skip top coats—who has the time? Besides, I don't need a top coat: I use Seche!

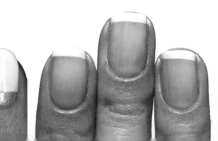

choosing a nail color

Here are some colors that look great with Latina skin tones:

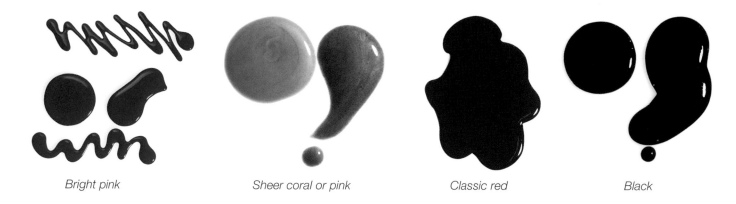

Bright pink *Sheer coral or pink* *Classic red* *Black*

faux nails

Fingernails are like orgasms: they shouldn't be faked. But I'd be lying if I told you I had never faked it—who hasn't been curious about acrylic tips and all those crazy designs you can do on them? I played a character in a soap opera who used fake nails. While I was shooting the soap, I had to use them for about a year. I got used to them, even grew to like them. But they got too long and switchblade-like, so I chopped them off. Later, when I went to Japan, fake nails were all the rage. What the Japanese were doing with fake nails was incredible. I ran out and got mine done right away! Leave it to the Japanese to turn fake nails into a fine art. They created fake nails with 3-D-like effects: flowers, rhinestones, stars, even lace. Since I couldn't bring a

Japanese nail salon back to the States with me, I settled for raiding the local drugstores for all their temporary press-on versions. I still have some packets at home.

When I am not reliving my stay in Japan, however, I wear my nails short and sweet. I prefer super-short square nails. Long nails age you, and repeated, long-term use of acrylic will weaken your natural nail. In a worst-case scenario, you could expose yourself to fungal infections if you don't keep up with the maintenance required. That said, I must admit that those press-on nails with funky designs and rhinestones are very cool for special, one-time use. But I recommend you stay away from the longer-term options.

nail-care tips

Here are some simple steps you can take to keep your nails looking marvelous.

✳ Keep a little pot of cuticle balm with you in your purse. I love Jing Jang Crème. It's a multiuse cream that can be applied to my nails or even my lips if they are chapped!

✳ Don't cut your cuticles, and don't let anyone else cut them, either. A regular manicure that includes a gentle

pushing back of the cuticles is all you need. Cuticles are like weeds. If they are cut, they grow back stronger.

✳ The most glamorous manicure option in my opinion? The French manicure. It's just more "jet set," has more cachet, and looks more polished than any other nail treatment.

best foot forward

A woman deserves feet that look sexy, pretty, and pampered year-round, whether she is sporting her household chanclas or teetering around in her strappy stilettos. Toenail polish goes a long way toward that goal. When I have public events, I stick to French pedicures, a classic red, or simple neutral colors. In my personal life, I go crazy: a different color for each toe, different designs for the big toe, or smiley-face and rhinestone appliqués. It's my secret eccentric side, my little pick-me-up. I have a nice surprise at the end of the day when I take off my Giuseppe Zanotti heels. But whether I'm keeping my toes simple or trying a crazy new design, I consider my weekly pedicure to be a vital part of my beauty routine. If you want fabulous pies, follow in my footsteps.

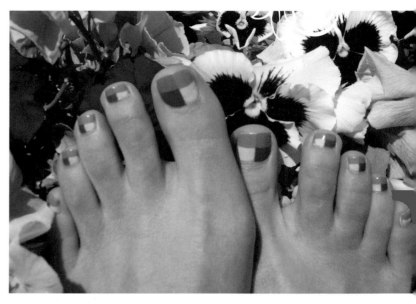

These are my toes and I had a great time getting this done just for fun, I couldn't stop looking down at them for a while.

pedicures

A professional pedicure is pampering at its best, but you can achieve many of the same effects at home.

✳ Remove nail polish with a gentle, nonacetone remover that won't dry your nails. Be sure to get the sides of the nails, where they meet the skin.

✳ Trim the nails with a high-quality clipper, trying to keep a consistent square shape.

✳ Apply a balm to the cuticles. I use a rich, multiuse cream. Submerge the feet in warm water for ten minutes. If you can add some marbles to the water, you will feel like you've just hired an expensive master masseuse for your feet: rub your feet over them for a maravilloso mini-massage. Make it a fun ritual. No marbles to play with? Try adding some soothing drops of lavender oil, or even rose petals for a visual effect.

✳ After their soak, scrub the feet and toenails with a soft-bristled nail brush. Rinse your feet with warm water and pat them dry.

✳ Use a foot file or pumice stone on the hard areas of the feet: the balls and heels, and even very gently on the tops of toes that have a tendency to callous.

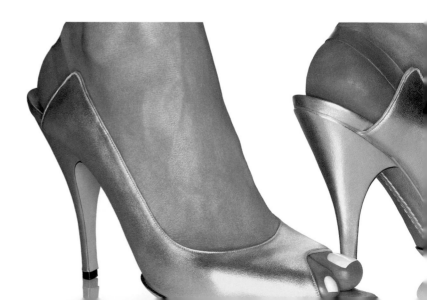

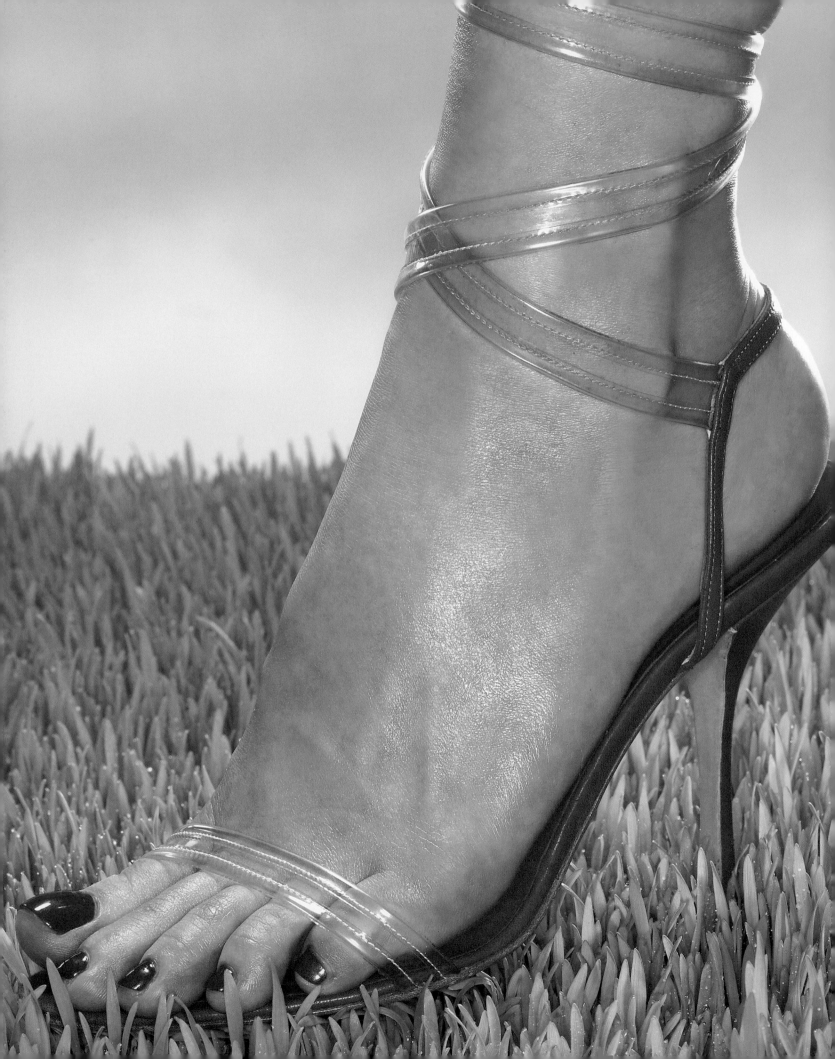

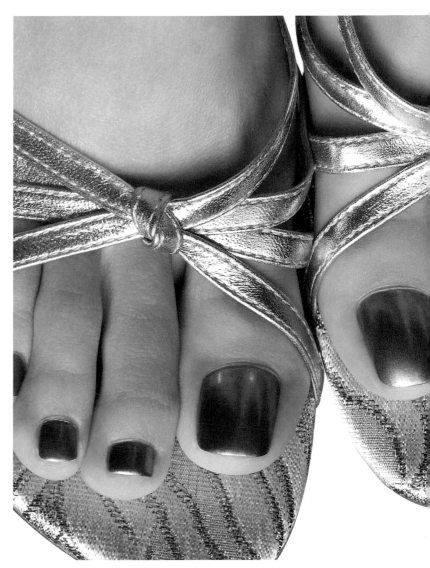

❊ Slather on a rich cream.

❊ Using nail polish remover and a cotton ball, wipe each nail clean of any oily residue. Make sure the nails are completely clean and dry.

❊ Gently push back the cuticles with a metal cuticle pusher with cotton wrapped around the tip.

❊ Use a foam toe separator to keep toes in place, and to keep your tiny pinky toe accessible.

❊ Apply a base coat. From base to tip, apply the coat first down the center of the nail, then on either side.

❊ Wait at least two minutes before applying color. As with your manicure, it may seem like an eternity, but it is worth the wait. Do a meditation on "beautiful, sexy feet." Apply a second coat.

❊ Skip the traditional top coat, and instead apply a fast-drying top coat.

❊ I end by applying a protective drying oil, which can help prevent nicks on the surface of the nail.

color cues and toe tips

As you can tell from my description of my crazy, funky pedicures, I'm not from the fingernails-must-match-toenails school of thought. I hate restrictive rules, and I think you should mix and match colors as you please. Here are some other thoughts on fierce-looking feet.

❊ No-fail toenail looks: a French pedicure (always fresh and youthful looking), a siren red (sexy!), a bright coral (best for bringing out your fabulous faux tan).

❊ A beauty treatment you can do in your sleep: Slather on a rich foot cream and the cuticle balm, pull on a pair of cotton socks, and hit the sack. You'll practically have new feet in the morning.

❊ A top coat keeps the pedicure looking fresh, especially after a day at the beach, when salt water and sand dull the shine. You can reapply the top coat every other day.

fabulous fragrance

My first fragrance was a baby cologne called Nenuco. My mami would apply it over my little body after my bath, before dressing me. From a very young age I associated fragrance with beauty, cleanliness, and being well cared for, which is why fragrance has become a personal passion of mine.

Fragrances are unique to each person. Two people applying the same fragrance on the same spot on their bodies at the same time will each "wear" the scent in different ways, because of individual body chemistry. Also, what a perfume smells like in the bottle may be nothing like what it smells like on your skin. This is why finding the right fragrance can sometimes be difficult. It's also tough to wade through all the different types of fragrances. Let me make it easy for you, so that the next time you are approached by a perfume salesperson and her spritzer, you won't skitter away in fear.

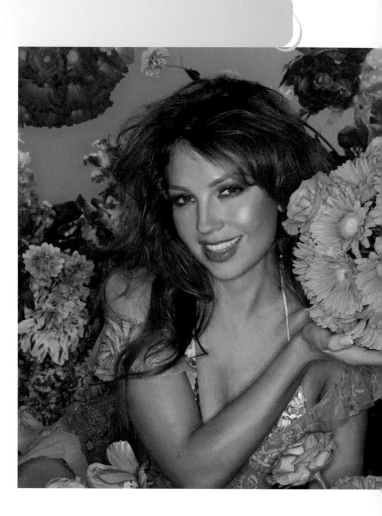

fragrance families

Different types of fragrances have different images and memories associated with them, which is one of the qualities that make a fragrance so personal. But understanding the types of fragrance available can also help you set your fragrance mood. Here are some fragrance families and the common scents most often associated with them:

WOODSY Sandalwood, oak, cedar

CITRUS Bergamot, lemon, orange, tangerine

FLORAL Gardenia, rose, lavender, jasmine

MUSK Patchouli, musk, ambergris

HERBAL Rosemary, sage, thyme

GREEN Grass, dewy leaves

cheat sheet on notes

Most perfumes are composed of three notes, each defined by how long the note will last.

TOP NOTE This is the first impression of a fragrance, what you smell immediately upon opening the bottle. It lasts fifteen minutes. Citrus or green scents are commonly used as top notes.

MIDDLE NOTE This is the essence of the fragrance, the scent that defines it. It surfaces five minutes after applying the fragrance to your skin.

BOTTOM NOTE This note surfaces after you have worn the fragrance for three to four hours.

types of fragrances

Ever wonder why you are charged $75 for an itty-bitty roll-on fragrance oil, but only $7.50 for a tub of after-bath splash? It has to do with the concentration of fragrance in the formula. Here is a primer on the different kinds of fragrances.

PERFUMES These have the highest ratio of pure fragrance oil to alcohol. Just a dab on a pulse point, such as your inner wrist, will leave you fragrant for hours. There is no need to layer a perfume with other products such as lotion, powder, or bubble bath, because the perfume should be potent enough on its own.

COLOGNE These are more diluted with alcohol than perfumes are. Cologne is the formula that works well with layering. Cologne also costs less than perfume, as you will notice at the store: a small bottle of eau de parfum costs more than a larger cologne-spray version of the same scent.

OILS These can be the most potent form of a fragrance; it depends on how much of the fragrant oil is mixed with the carrier oil. I like oils, especially in the winter. There is something more sensual about them.

BODY SPLASHES This formulation has the lowest concentration of pure fragrance or essential oils. Splashes are great in summer, because they are bracing and refreshing. The downside: by the end of the day, no trace of their fragrance remains.

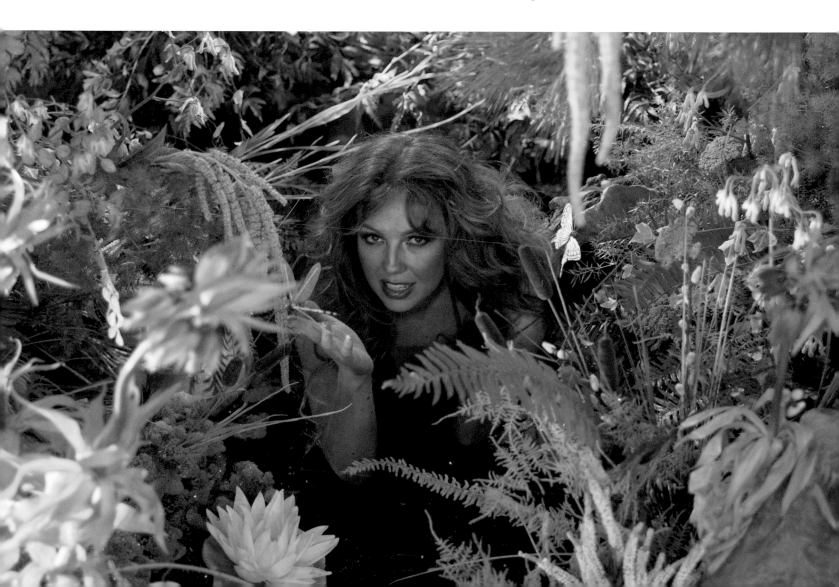

how to buy a fragrance

Most fragrances are not cheap, so keeping these tips in mind will help you make the best decision next time you approach the perfume counter.

❋ If you see coffee beans at the counter, take a whiff between fragrances. The beans are meant to clear your head, so you do not confuse one fragrance with another.

❋ Use blotter papers: spray the fragrance liberally on a paper to get a sense of the scent on its own, apart from your body chemistry. Once you have narrowed the choices down to no more than three, spray one on each wrist and the third on the inside of your elbow.

❋ Remember what I explained about top notes and bottom notes? Wait at least fifteen minutes, smell the spritzed spots again, and then make a decision about which fragrance to select.

❋ Ask for a sample and wear it for a few days.

❋ A great scent should lift your mood and boost your confidence. If it doesn't, then it is simply not worth the money. Only go with a fragrance that does something for you.

❋ We all have become fans of the red-carpet shots of celebrities. I certainly love to look at them! If you have a designer whose garments you tend to admire— say you love the sexy, colorful Cavalli or the regal, elegant lines of Carolina Herrera—you might want to try the designer's fragrance, because it will have been created to convey that designer's signature style via scent instead of fabric, cut, and color.

spritz tips

The best time to apply fragrance is in the morning, after you have showered and applied your body lotion, but before you dress. Most women tend to put on perfume after they have dressed and right before they run out the door, but that makes it hard to apply to the primary spots that keep a fragrance vivid throughout the day: the pulse points. Starting from the bottom and working upward, spray the ankles, the navel, the base of the neck, the upper part of the neck just behind the ears, and the inner wrists. Some women also like to spritz their inner elbows and even their cleavage.

layering and gender bending

Back in the day, I was the queen of layering fragrances. I went through my Thierry Mugler's Angel phase. I'd take a bath in it, moisturize my skin with it, and then spritz it on my wrists and neck before leaving the house. I did the same with Samba by Liz Claiborne and Poison by Dior. Layering—using a fragrance in its soap or bath gel, body cream, and perfume or cologne form—is great when you want to really luxuriate in the scent itself, and don't mind asphyxiating your boyfriend and innocent passers-by as you waft along, oblivious to the fact that they smell you before they see you. Today I prefer to apply a strong scent very sparingly: I will spray some on a tissue and gently dust the Kleenex over my neck and décolletage. Or I will spray a puff into the air and allow the scent to envelope me in a light mist.

I also like to mix different scents, and I don't worry about fragrance clash—that's an old-fashioned idea that went out with having to match your toenail color with your fingernail color. When I layer now, I usually mix fragrance oils, the ones that come in the tiny roller-ball vials. I literally double-apply two different vials (an Egyptian musk with a sandalwood, for example) to my wrists and behind my ears. My favorite fragrance oils are by Carol's Daughter. They last all day and they are small enough for me to throw in my purse if I am feeling like I want a midday fragrance boost.

But for really gutsy layering, men's fragrances are the undiscovered gold mine. I love men's fragrances so much I wear them myself! Men's fragrances are strong and bold, never timid and apologetic, which is how some women's fragrances strike me. Some of my favorites are Chanel's Égoiste, and Lowes.

aromatherapy

I was skeptical that applying a mix of lavender oil to my temples would stop a migraine until I actually tried it for myself. Since then I have been a believer, and I use aromatherapy principles to help me get energized, to relax me at night, and to focus when I need to concentrate on a task at hand. Aromatherapy practices go back hundreds, if not thousands, of years. They are based on the principle that certain scents can be healing, soothing, even energizing.

Calming scents: chamomile, sage, jasmine, lemon balm
Energizing scents: eucalyptus, lemon, orange, ginger

The Body Shop is a great source for ready-mixed aromatherapy blends, but if you are in a DIY state of mind, here is a recipe that you can use with a ceramic candle diffuser to create a calm atmosphere in the evening. Make this mixture to add to the bowl of the diffuser. It uses the essential oils of sweet orange, ylang-ylang, and lavender. You can purchase essential oils at health food stores.

* 1 to 2 tablespoons water

* 4 drops essential oil of sweet orange

* 2 drops essential oil of ylang-ylang

* 1 drop essential oil of lavender

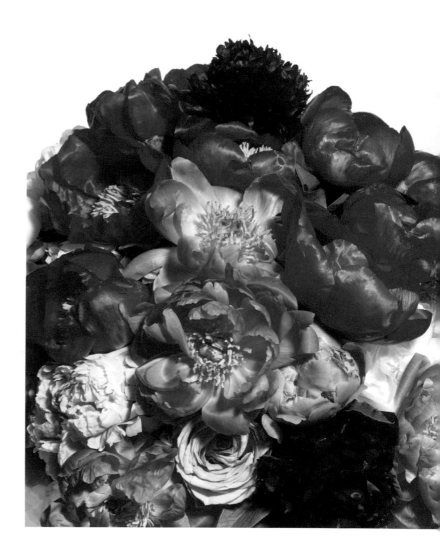

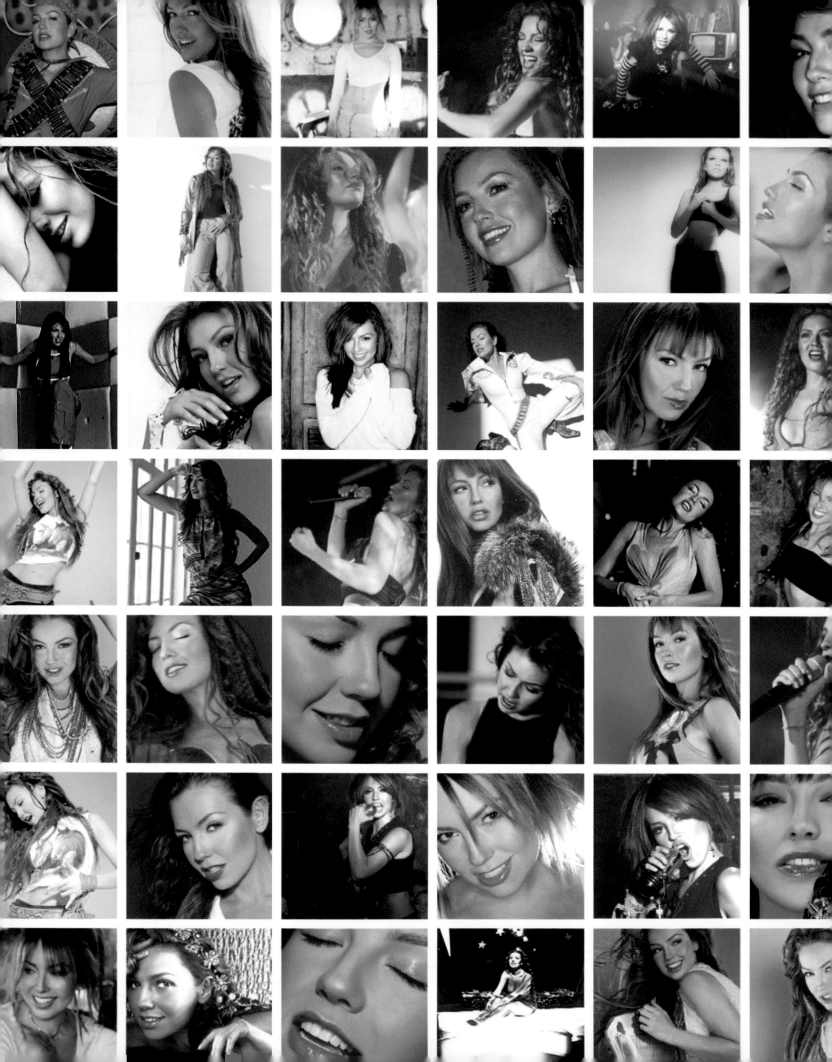

glamorama

DIFFERENT LOOKS

As you can tell from the previous pages, I have experimented with *many* different looks throughout my career. While it would be impossible for me to take you through every single look, I can tell you this: I love change and taking risks. If I didn't, I never would have come to America. I had a great life in Mexico, but I wanted to explore, try new things, and push myself. It's the urge we all have to reinvent ourselves and challenge people's perceptions of us. That dare-to-be-different attitude is what this chapter is all about. What I love the most about hair, makeup, and fashion is the potential for total transformation.

There are a ton of different looks here to inspire you. Some of them are for day-to-day wear. Others are for big-night-out extravaganzas. Some of the changes are easy. Other changes required a whole team of experts to help me execute. But I'm keeping the steps as simple as possible so that you can achieve this at home. We did it all: wigs, extensions, crazy false lashes, and even body makeup. Try the entire look or just a part of it—it's up to you.

glamazon bombshell

The bronzer, the better, in this no-sun-damage yet beautifully brown look. Try it for a hot summer night.

FACE AND BODY

✳ Apply foundation and concealer to even your skin tone.

✳ Use foundation sponges to apply and blend a liquid bronzer on the cheeks, forehead, and chin to give the skin an allover glow. Liquid bronzer is the best option in this case, because you want the skin to remain as fresh and touchable-looking as possible. If you are more comfortable with powder bronzers, build the color with each application.

✳ When you think you are through blending, blend some more. Whenever you are making a change in skin tone as dramatic as this one, it is critical that you blend.

✳ Extend the bronzer to your décolletage, your bare back (get your honey to help you; think of it as cosmetically enhanced foreplay), and your shoulders. The end effect will be as though you are bathed in radiance.

CHEEKS

✳ Use a neutral-toned gel blush to give a subtle color to the apples of your cheeks. Gel blush, like cream blush, is better for looks—like this one—that are not matte or heavy.

✳ Use your fingers to pat the color onto your cheeks.

✳ As with the bronzer, blend, blend, blend—this time working quickly, because the gel formula dries rapidly.

EYES

✳ The eyes create the smolder factor in this look, but instead of doing a traditional gray, smoky eye, use tones of copper, gold, and bronze to create a golden-hued—yet still smoky—eye.

✳ Use the gold as a base color, the copper to contour, and a bronze shadow with a pearlescent formula along the upper and lower lash line.

✳ Because this look is so strong, add individual bunches of false lashes along the outer thirds of your top lash line.

✳ Finish with a coat of black or brown mascara.

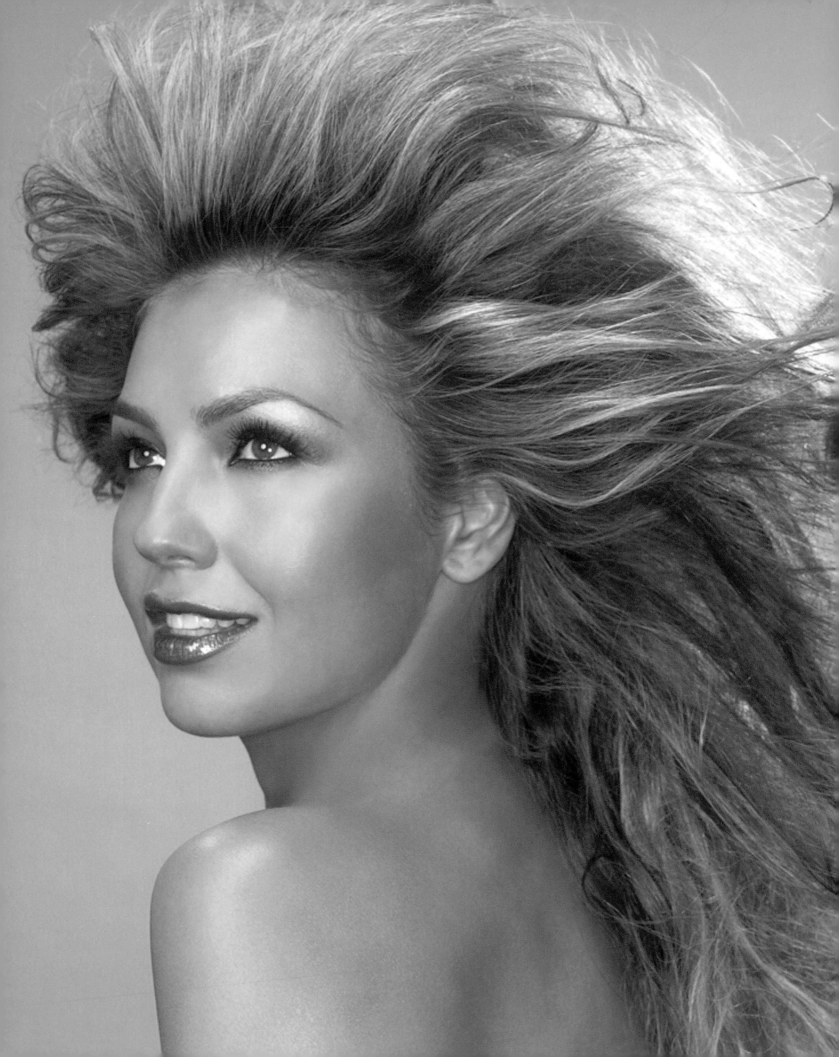

LIPS

✳ The lips here are strong in order to ensure that they do not become washed out in the midst of such a sun-drenched look.

✳ Use neutral colors to create a strong, defined lip look. Select a skin-tone-colored or slightly darker brown lip-liner. Apply it along the lip line and fill your lips with the liner, for lasting color.

✳ Apply a bronzed gold lip color over your lips with a lip brush.

HAIR

✳ Add extensions in various lowlights and highlights to create this amped-up, glorious mane. Start with dry hair.

✳ Tease your hair at the crown with a rat-tailed comb and use lots of hair spray.

✳ Use strategically placed bobby pins to not only secure the extensions along the sides and back of your head, but also to create a frame at the crown to help pump up the volume.

✳ Apply more hair spray when you have secured the extensions. It will be critical to keeping your hold, because this hairstyle defies gravity.

Takeaway tip: Bronzer gives a glistening warmth, but be sure to blend well.

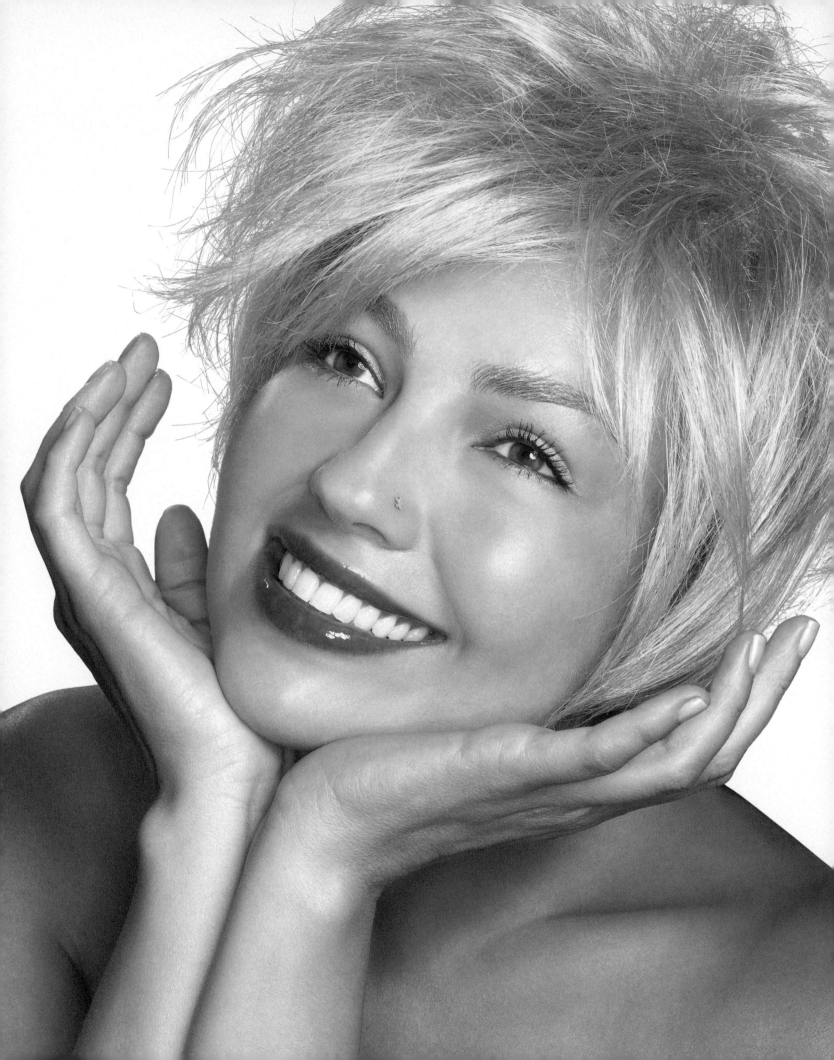

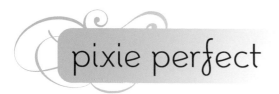

pixie perfect

Have you ever donned a wig? It's amazing, the different persona it can bring out. Try wearing one for a party or out to a club.

FACE

❋ Apply a light coating of foundation with a dampened sponge only where needed.

❋ Use concealer lightly and only in areas of discoloration, such as under your eyes or around the nose and mouth.

❋ To give this look un tu que mas, use eyelash glue to attach a tiny rhinestone as a faux nose ring.

CHEEKS

❋ If you always use powder blush, try a cream blush to get a long-lasting glow from within.

❋ Apply the blush on the apples of your cheeks and blend well for a slightly flushed look.

EYES

❋ Choose a light, sheer, brightly colored eye shadow with just a hint of shimmer in the formula to brighten the eyes.

❋ Don't use eyeliner or fake lashes. Just curl your lashes with an eyelash curler and apply a light coating of mascara, to make sure the eyes do not disappear.

❋ Tweeze, comb, and apply gel to your brows, but no powder or liner are needed.

❋ Apply a coat of eyebrow color in a shade or two lighter than your natural color.

LIPS

❋ No lip-liner needed here, just an application of a sheer berry gloss.

HAIR

❋ Try a wig in a pixie-style haircut.

❋ Keep in mind that even if you are experimenting with a dramatic change in hair length and color (even with a wig, like I did here), you don't need to camouflage your face with tons of makeup. A short hairstyle can be very feminine and flirty—and yes, very sexy!

Takeaway tip: This look is proof that less is more. Especially if you want to look younger, you have to keep things fun yet simple. Dewy, clean makeup that lets your skin show through is the goal.

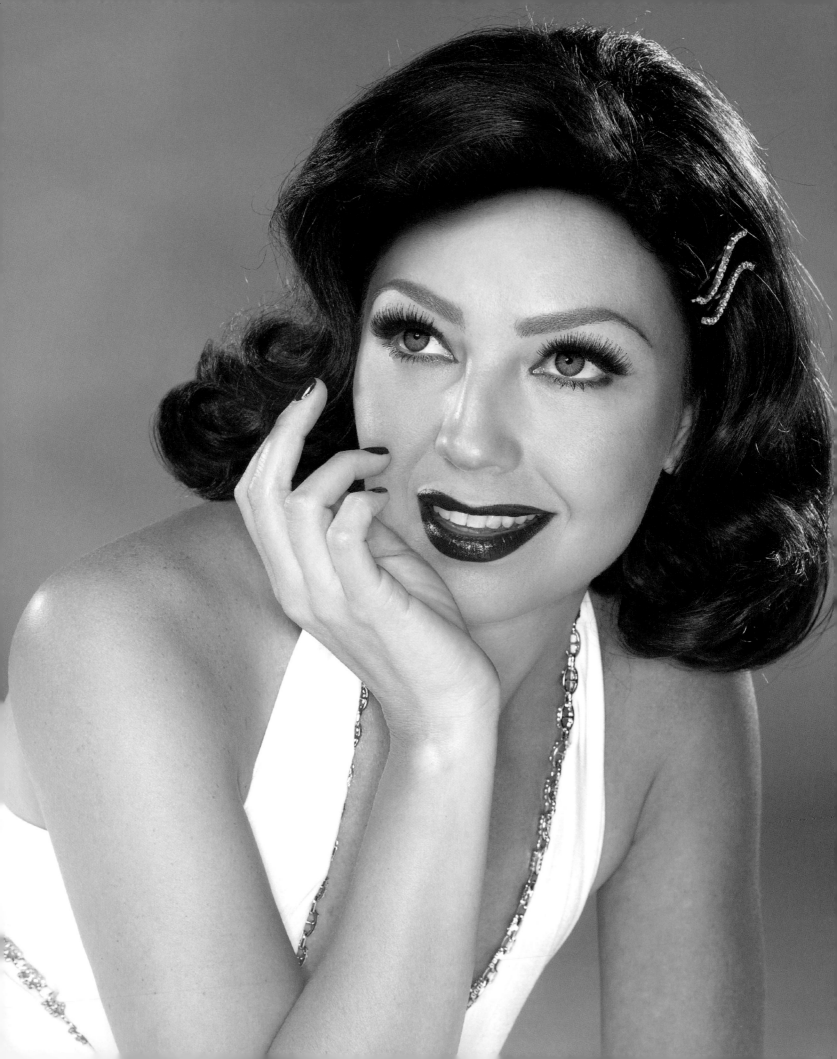

screen siren

This is my homage to Elizabeth Taylor, one of my favorite old-school actresses.

FACE

❋ Smooth, porcelain skin was the look of the 1950s, so use matte foundation to even your skin tone completely.

❋ Use concealer around your eyes and nose to perfect the canvas.

❋ Apply a light dusting of loose translucent powder to set your foundation and smooth your skin.

CHEEKS

❋ Dust the apples of your cheeks with a rose-pink powder blush. Using a blush brush, blend the color back and upward to accentuate your cheekbones and avoid looking severe.

EYES

❋ Prepare a base for your eye shadow with a golden, slightly iridescent eye shadow applied from the lash line to the brow bone.

❋ Use a slightly darker—but only slightly darker—color to contour the crease of your eye. Keep the shadows simple, because the eyeliner will be heavy.

❋ Apply a thin application of liquid eyeliner along your entire upper lash line.

❋ To create a thicker outer line, draw a second line only on the outer third of your upper lash line. Extend the line slightly to create a dramatic effect.

❋ Use eyeliner pencil along the lower lash line and inner eyes.

❋ Apply a strip of false eyelashes for a final eye-opening effect.

LIPS

❋ Prep your lips by gently exfoliating and applying a nongreasy lip balm.

❋ Apply concealer around the lips to even out your skin tone in the area.

❋ Use a red lip-liner to line and fill in your lips. This will prevent "bleeding" of the lip color and will help it last longer.

❋ Use a lip brush and apply an iconic, classic red such as MAC's Russian Red (which I used here), an ultrabright blue-red color that flatters a wide range of skin tones.

HAIR

❋ Use rollers to create alluring old-school waves.

❋ I wanted to use auburn hair for this look. That hair color choice informed my makeup choices. Darker hair demands that you use a blush that will keep the rest of your face from washing out.

Takeaway tip: If you like this look, try the voluminous false eyelashes—you'll instantly feel like a Hollywood starlet.

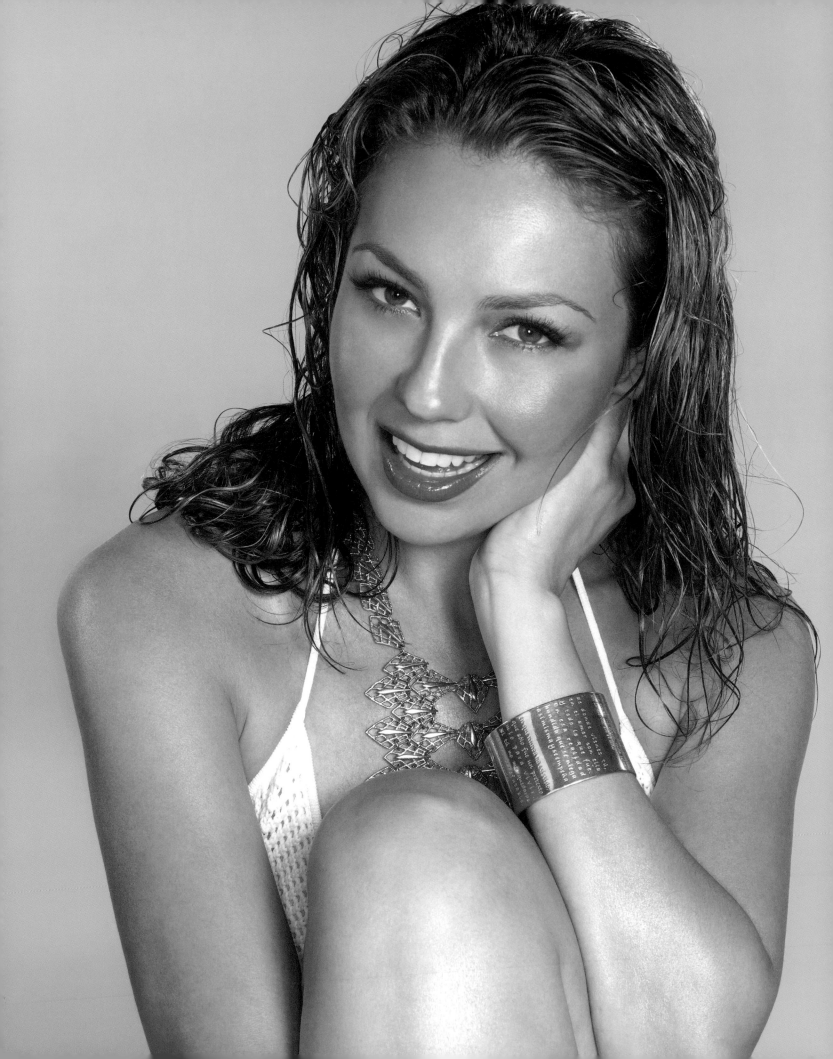

st. tropez

This look will give you fresh, touchable skin and hair. This is a beach or poolside look that is easy on the eyes and easy to achieve. ¡Súper fresco!

FACE AND BODY

✳ Apply concealer only to the areas that need it, such as the folds of your nose and the area around the mouth. You may find that you can skip foundation altogether if you don't need any.

✳ For vibrant, luminous-looking skin, use a sheer foundation to even out any discoloration.

✳ Make sure that the skin on your body is hydrated and moisturized. Apply a lotion with a slight shimmer to your chest, arms, and legs.

CHEEKS

✳ Apply a cream blush to the apples of your cheeks to create an outdoorsy flush.

✳ Blend it well with your fingertips, getting it to almost melt into your skin for a seamless, radiant sheen.

EYES

✳ Keep it super-simple. Apply a pearlescent copper eye shadow around the lash line.

✳ Apply a few groups of false lashes with a waterproof lash glue to the outer lash line.

✳ Curl the lashes with an eyelash curler.

✳ Apply waterproof mascara with a light touch, to blend the false eyelashes with your own and to give length to the tips.

✳ Tweeze and brush the brows, then seal them with a clear gel to keep them in place.

LIPS

✳ Apply a cherry-toned gloss to give your face a splash of color.

✳ If you like, choose a high-shine formula to give the illusion of full, pillowy lips.

HAIR

✳ Dampen your hair with water, then apply styling cream to prevent frizz.

✳ In a real beach situation, use a styling cream with an SPF or apply a conditioning mask, to protect your hair from the harsh sun and salt water.

Takeaway tip: Beach-ready beauty means a flash of color on the lips and cheeks—iy listo!

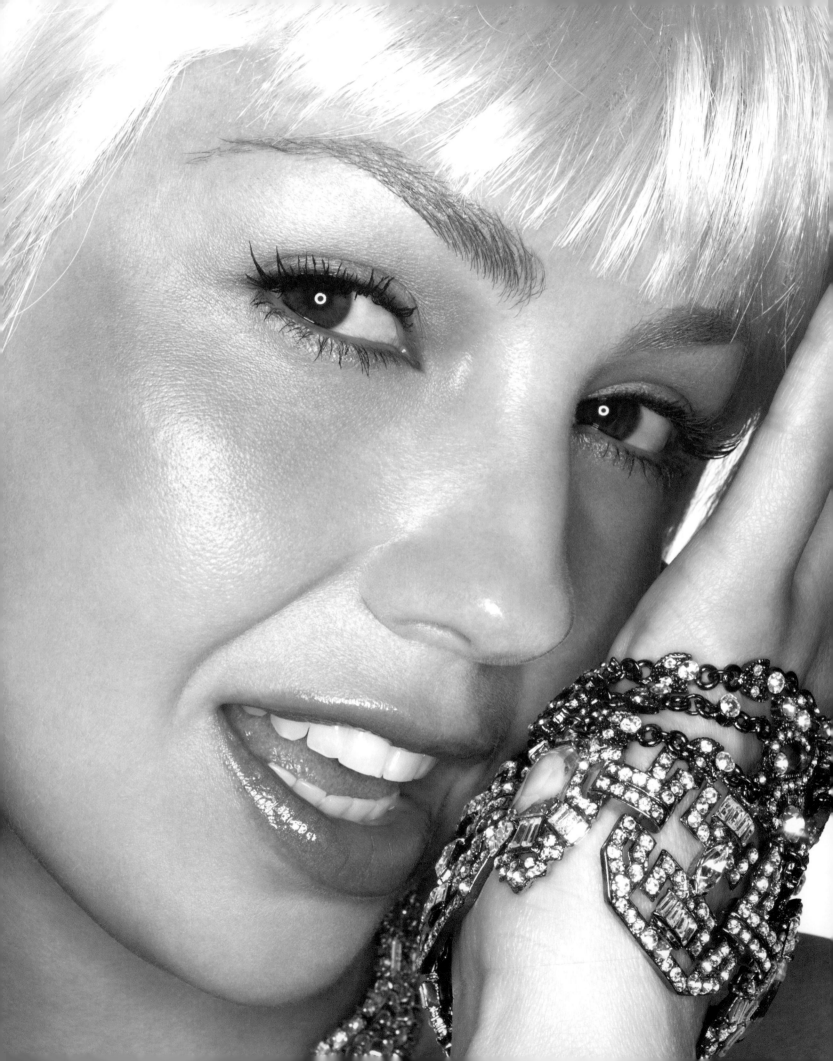

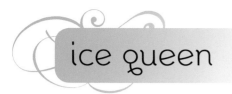

ice queen

A flapper-era bob, deceptively simple makeup, and accessories with bling give this retro look a modern twist. It's a youthful style that anyone can adopt.

FACE

❋ Moisturize the face for a healthy glow.

❋ Lightly apply a sheer foundation to minimize imperfections without heavy, opaque coverage.

❋ Skip the powder: for this look you want to see the skin.

CHEEKS

❋ Use a cream blush in a bright pink shade. Apply it in layers with your fingers. Build the color slowly, because too much will have a clown effect.

❋ Apply a light, pearlescent highlighter to the upper apples of the cheeks to bump up your skin's glow.

EYES

❋ This is a simple eye look. Apply a sheer wash of lavender cream eye shadow on the lid, from the lash line to the brow bone. The lavender color choice really makes the eyes pop.

❋ An iridescent green eyeliner along the lower and inner lash line brings even more color into the mix.

❋ Skip the liner and fake lashes.

❋ Apply one coat of mascara to ensure that the lashes won't be lost in the eye color. Be sure to use only one coat, because any more than that would look too heavy-handed.

LIPS

❋ Such soft eyes and cheeks can be paired with a defined lip. Use a dusty-pink lip-liner to define the lip line and fill in the color.

❋ Over the liner, apply a sheer lip gloss in a crushed raspberry color to give the lips a sheen of pigment.

HAIR

❋ Cut a platinum-blonde wig into a bob at a symmetrical angle along your jawline—higher in the back and longer as it angles in the front—to flatter and frame the face.

❋ Platinum-blonde bobs are usually paired with heavy, dramatic makeup. Here I've shown you that a different approach still works.

Takeaway tip: Experiment with color on the eyes, lips, and cheeks by using sheer, blendable colors that won't look too heavy or clownish.

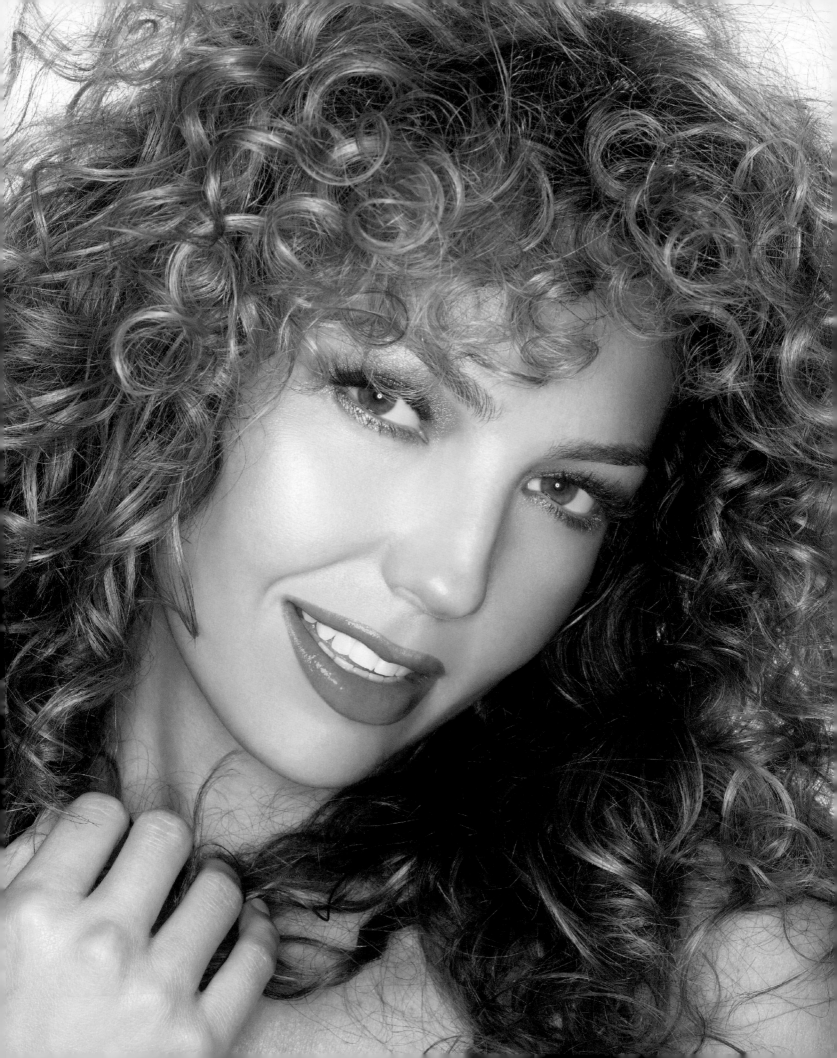

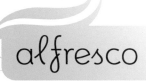

alfresco

A frame of curls and cherubic cheeks make this another youthful look that will flatter any face. This look is great for weekends.

FACE

❊ Apply a liquid foundation for smooth, even-textured skin.

❊ Use concealer around the eyes, nose, and mouth to create a creamy, even-toned surface.

❊ Set the base with a light dusting of loose translucent powder.

CHEEKS

❊ Think of old-fashioned rouge: use a cream blush in dusty pink on the apples of the cheeks to give a hint of color.

❊ Blend with your fingertips to extend the flush upward and outward.

EYES

❊ On the ball of the lid apply a yellow eye shadow with golden flecks to draw light to the eye.

❊ Apply pinkish copper highlights on the brow bone.

❊ For contour, a deeper rum color shapes the crease of the eye.

❊ Apply a deeper shimmery copper eyeliner along the lower lash line.

LIPS

❊ Soft, kissable lips are the goal. Gently line the lip with a pinkish-brown lip-liner.

❊ Add color with a creamy pink lip gloss for a smooth luster.

HAIR

❊ Start with dry hair. Use a small-barrel curling iron to create slender, angelic curls.

❊ Separate each curl into two or more individual curls to create a massive mane of tiny corkscrews.

❊ Apply only a quick spritz of hair spray to keep the shape of the curls. Anything heavier would weigh the curls down.

Takeaway tip: Vivacious, rowdy ringlets and curlicues keep their shape best with a light-holding hair spray.

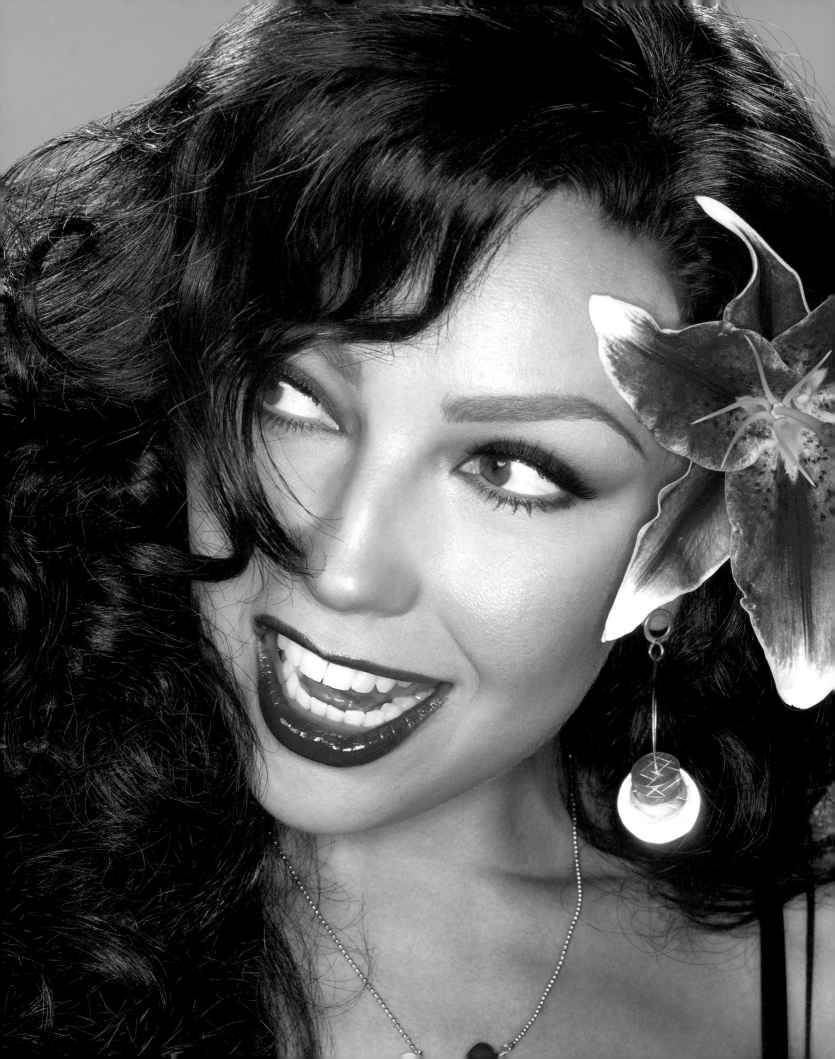

old-school latina

This is an homage to the feisty '50s screen icons from old cine Mexicano, like María Felix and Dolores Del Rio.

FACE

✻ Use matte foundation to even the skin tone completely, minimize pores, and create a flawless surface.

✻ Apply concealer around the eyes, nose, and anywhere else with darker pigmentation.

✻ Use a light dusting of loose translucent powder to set the foundation. Remember to use only one light application, because too much powder is aging and becomes cakey.

CHEEKS

✻ Dust the apples of the cheeks with a peachy-rose powder blush.

✻ Using a blush brush, blend backward and upward to accentuate the cheekbones, but avoid looking severe.

✻ Place a dot of highlighter on the tops of the cheeks and blend well over the blush. This gives a sheen and prevents the makeup from looking too mattelike.

EYES

✻ Prepare the base of the eye by applying a golden matte eye shadow from the lash line to the brow bone.

✻ Use a matte dark brown to contour in the crease of the eye.

✻ Apply a dark gray matte shadow on the ball of the lid and along the top lash line.

✻ Using a sharpened black eyeliner pencil, draw a thin line along the entire upper lash line.

✻ Use the pencil to draw a line along the bottom lash line, thickening the line ever so slightly on the outer eye.

✻ Apply a strip of false eyelashes for a final eye-opening effect.

✻ Brows should be groomed and strong, but not overly done.

LIPS

✻ Prep the lips by gently exfoliating and then moisturizing with a nongreasy lip balm.

✻ Apply concealer around the lips to even out the skin tone in that area.

✻ Use a lip-liner that matches your skin tone to line and fill in the lips.

✻ Using a lip brush, apply red lipstick. Cover with a clear, shiny gloss to keep from looking too dated.

HAIR

✻ I am wearing a wig in this shot. To create soft, feminine curls, use hot rollers on your hair.

✻ Wearing a coquettish, bright flower in your hair gives a romantic edge to your whole look.

Takeaway tip: Don't shy away from bold makeup paired with other strong colors.

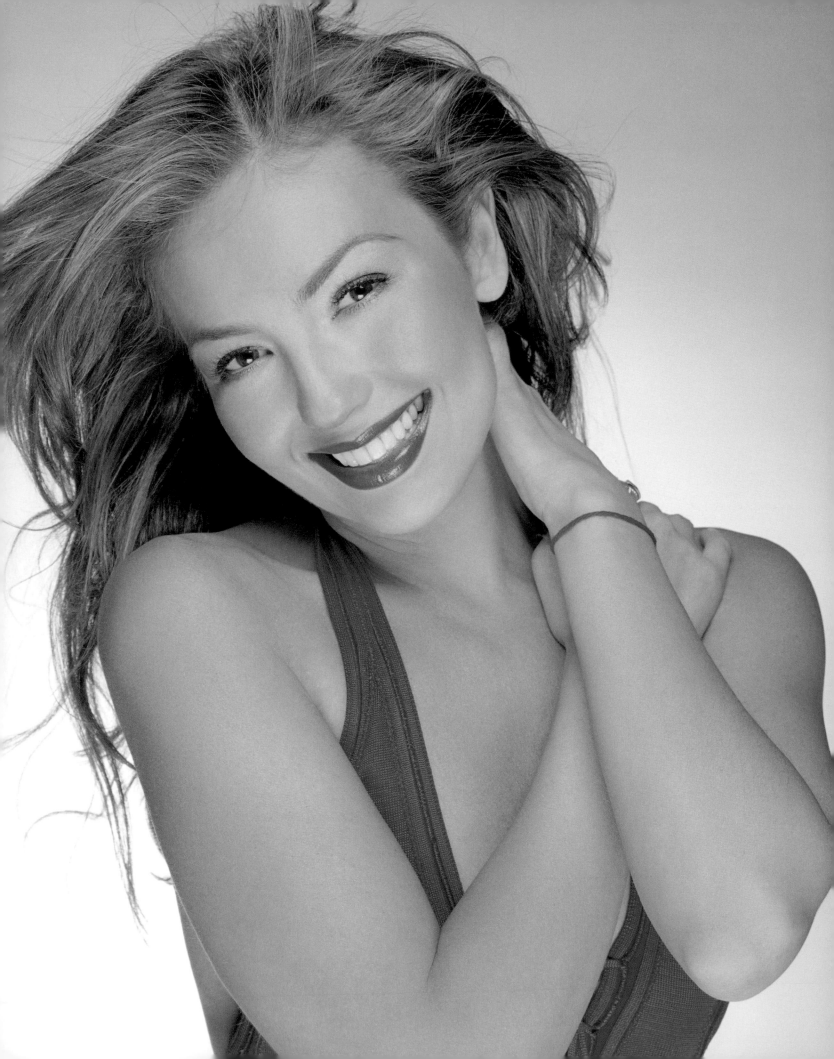

new millennium latina

This look will take you from the office to after-work drinks. It is fresh and bold, just like us Latinas.

FACE

❋ With a damp makeup sponge for maximum blendability, apply foundation.

❋ Use illuminating concealer under the eyes and in the inner corners of the eyes, to draw light and open the area.

❋ Smooth any blemishes or bumps with regular concealer.

CHEEKS

❋ With a fluffy brush, apply a soft pink powder blush on the cheeks, which will complement the lips without making everything too bright or overdone.

EYES

❋ The focus of this look is the lips, so the eye color is somewhat muted. Apply an iridescent, almost white shadow as a base color from the lash line to the brow bone.

❋ Add depth with a neutral brown color in the crease, and blend upward into the brow bone.

❋ Apply a very thin line of copper eye shadow or pencil along the top and bottom lash line. Keep the line thin, and don't extend it beyond the eye. For this look, you don't want drama in the eyes.

❋ A squeeze on the eyelash curler, a swipe of mascara, and the eyes are done.

LIPS

❋ This is a modern update to the siren-red lips usually associated with the typical "Latina" look. Instead of heavy matte lipstick, it uses a shiny, high-gloss, lacquered look. First, line and fill the lips with a lip-liner as close to your natural lip color as possible.

❋ With a lip brush, apply a rich red lipstick in a cream blush formula or a 24-hour stain-proof formula.

❋ On top of that, apply a coat of clear, high-shine gloss. My favorite is Lip Glass by MAC. This will give you a modern update on the siren red.

HAIR

❋ Blow-dry your hair straight for smoothness.

❋ Use a round brush to shape the ends, to keep body and movement.

❋ Create volume at the crown with a root volumizer.

Takeaway tip: Red lips are an anywhere, anytime beauty classic.

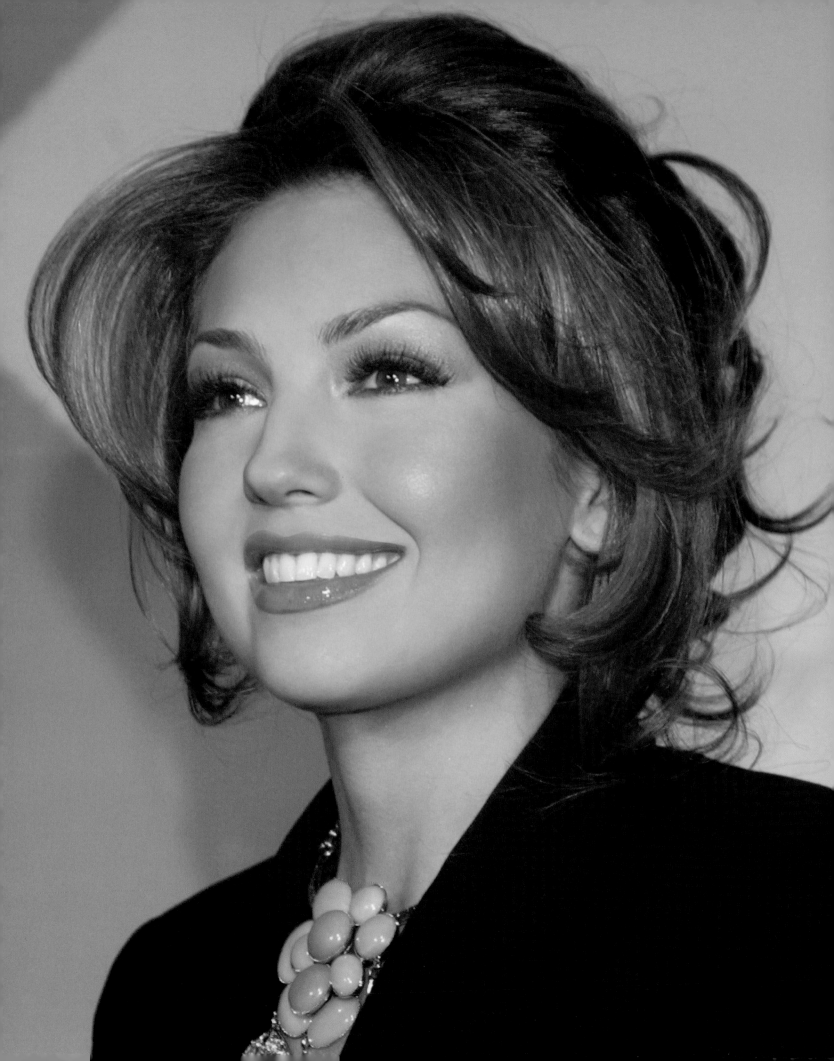

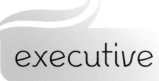

executive

Makeup that stays on all day is a necessity, but the color choices in this look have to convey an "easy and approachable" personality. This makeup is a must for the boardroom.

FACE

❋ Apply a matte foundation in a nondrying formula.

❋ Blend it with a damp sponge, going for even coverage all over the face.

❋ Seal with a light coating of translucent powder to set the makeup.

CHEEKS

❋ Apply a neutral peachy-brown blush on the apples of the cheeks for a wash of color.

❋ The end result should be a wash of color that won't fade as the day goes by.

EYES

❋ Use soft colors that still define and shape the eye. On the lid, apply a base color in a neutral taupe or beige, in a light cream formula, to hold longer.

❋ A soft walnut-brown powder shadow, applied to the crease of your eye as a contour, will adhere beautifully to the cream shadow underneath for a look that will last for hours.

❋ With a soft brown eyeliner, draw a line along the lash line of the upper lid. Use a Q-tip to soften and blend the line into the shadow.

❋ Curl the eyelashes and end with an application of mascara for wide, alert eyes (false eyelashes optional).

LIPS

❋ Use neutral colors to create a strong, defined lip look. A skin-tone or pink lip-liner is a good choice. Apply it along the lip line and fill the lips with the liner, for lasting color.

❋ Apply a creamy dusty-pink lip color over the lips.

❋ Blot the lips with a tissue before reapplying a second coat of lipstick to ensure smooth wear throughout the day.

HAIR

❋ A flowing up-do is serious without seeming too severe. Pull the longer hair in back into a loose chignon, secured with bobby pins and hair spray.

❋ Style the hair around the face and on the sides in face-framing wisps using a round brush and a blow-dryer, almost to suggest the look of a shorter hairstyle.

❋ For bangs that are layered and soft, but not unkempt, prep them with gel for a soft yet lasting hold, then style them with a round brush and blow-dryer.

Takeaway tip: For long-wearing lip color, use a creamy or matte formula with staying power. Avoid gloss.

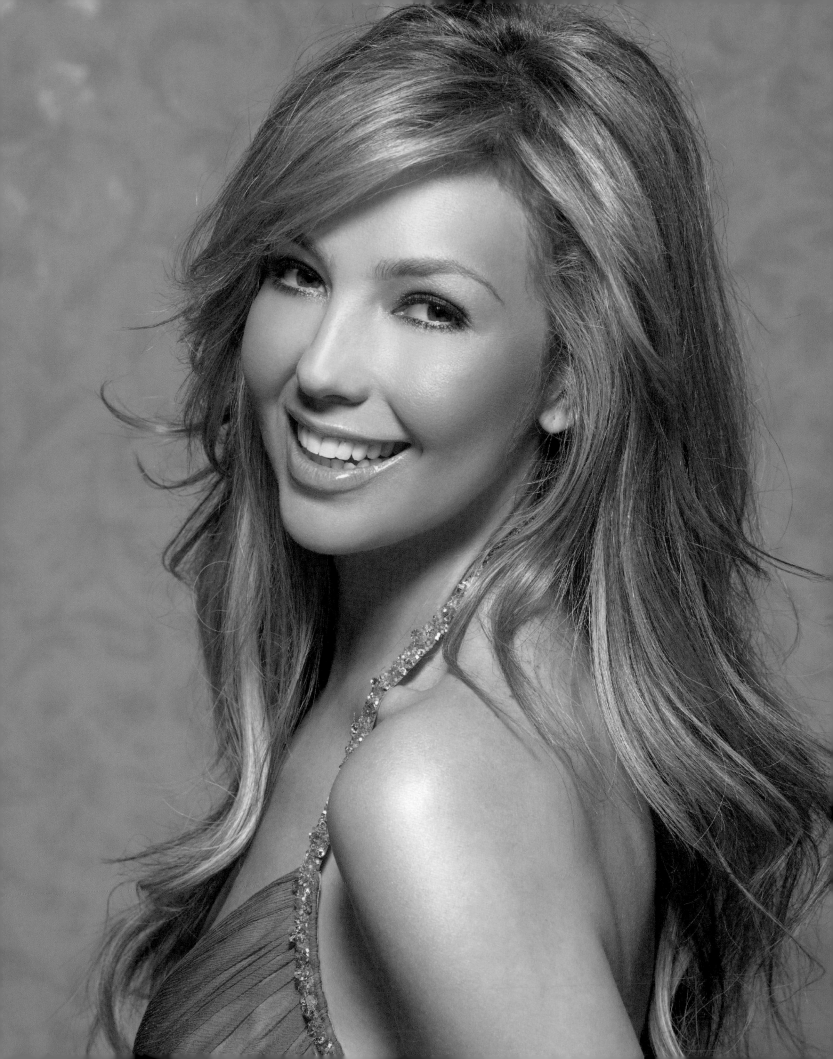

young hollywood

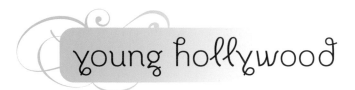

This look will make you red-carpet ready (or salsa-club scintillating) in a flash!

FACE AND BODY

❋ Skin is in for this look, so a sheer, luminous base that enhances, not covers, the skin is what you are going for. Apply a sheer foundation to even the skin tone and blend it well, for a flawless look.

❋ Apply an illuminating concealer to the under-eye area.

❋ Skip the matte powder. Instead, apply a loose iridescent powder. Apply the powder generously over the décolletage and shoulders as well. You should look like you have been dipped in honey.

CHEEKS

❋ Apply highlighter on the tops of the cheeks and at the tip of the nose, to add a sheen to the skin.

❋ Use a cream or gel blush in a neutral color for a soft flush that looks like it emanates from within.

❋ Blend the blush and highlighter well, using your fingertips to warm the makeup onto the skin.

EYES

❋ For the lid color, stick to a neutral shade in a high-sparkle formula.

❋ The contour shadow is the most important: apply a high-shine yet darker-toned eye shadow in the hollows of the crease and blend upward toward the brow bone.

❋ Apply the highlighter to the brow bone and also to the inner eyes, to really brighten and open up the eyes.

❋ Curl your eyelashes and be generous with the mascara for a coqueto, curly look.

LIPS

❋ Line the lips with a skin-toned pencil for lushness and definition, but make the line soft by blending it into the lips with your finger.

❋ Top with a shimmery nude gloss, to give a hint of color and a lot of shine.

HAIR

❋ Blow-dry the hair straight, for smoothness. Use a large-barrel curling iron for a soft wavy effect.

❋ Apply volumizing spray to the roots at the crown.

❋ Use a wide-tooth comb to smooth the top layers of the hair back.

❋ Spray with a high-sheen-formula hair spray to keep the mile-high halo from falling.

Takeaway tip: Amp up your skin's natural glow with a generous application of glittery body powder whenever you wear a skin-baring outfit.

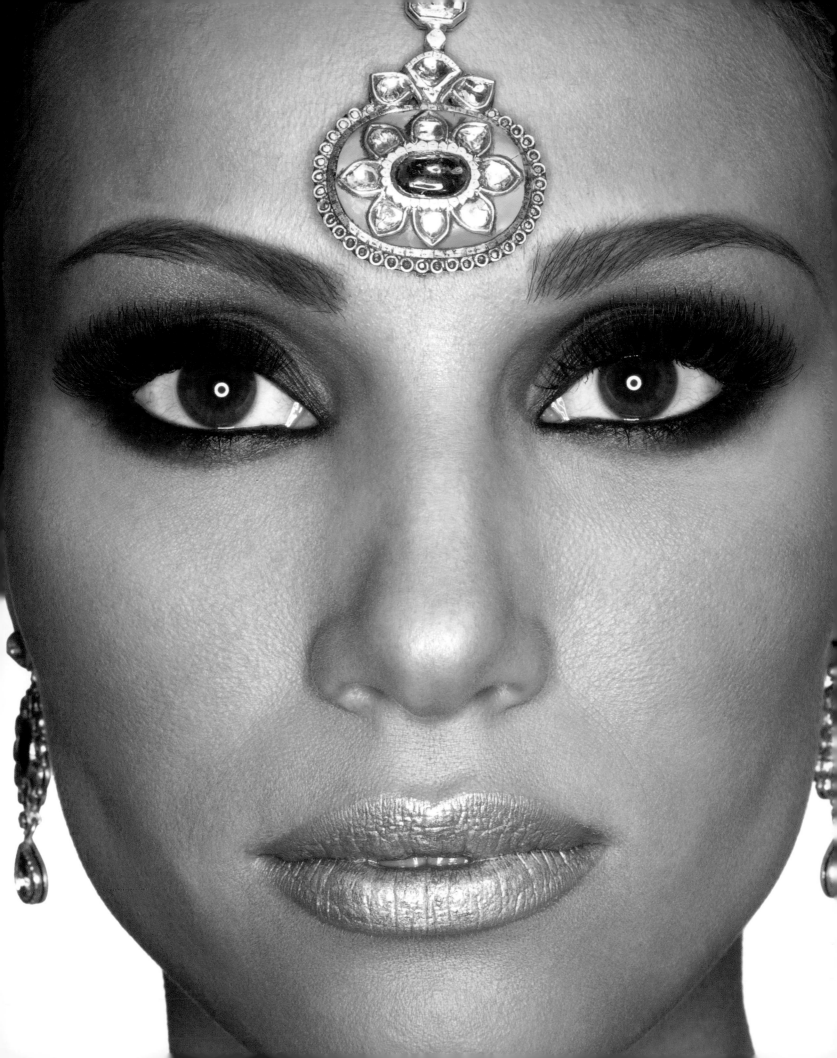

bollywood

Flawless skin with a honey-toned glow is paired with exotic eyes in this enticing look, which is great for a night out.

FACE

❃ Apply a foundation to smooth the canvas and prepare the skin.

❃ Around the eyes, go extra-light with the concealer. Use only the amount necessary to cover up the dark areas. Any excess concealer will cake into the fine lines of this look's heavy eye makeup.

❃ Apply a light dusting of loose translucent powder to set the makeup.

CHEEKS

❃ Contouring and highlighting shape the face in this look. Apply contour to the hollows of the cheeks, along the jawline and the sides of the nose, and at the temples.

❃ Apply highlighter along the tops of the cheeks, down the center of the nose, and on the chin.

❃ Blend, blend, blend with a damp makeup sponge.

EYES

❃ Prepare the eye area with an eye-shadow base, which will hold the shadow and prevent creasing.

❃ Start with a small eye-shadow brush and apply a dark gray shadow to the lid, starting from the lash line and blending up toward the crease. Apply in layers, building the color gradually.

❃ Blend the shadow upward and outward.

❃ Use the small brush to slowly apply a thick line of the gray shadow along the upper and lower lash lines. Circle the eye completely, to mimic the effect of Indian kohl liner.

❃ Because the lashes can get lost in the shadow, apply a strip of false lashes along the upper lash line. Apply a second shorter strip from mid-eye to outer eye.

LIPS

❃ The overpowering eyes here demand a light lip, so skip the lip-liner and go straight to the gloss.

❃ Apply a creamy–not glittery–gloss in a neutral color. This will ensure the lips do not disappear into the face, but won't distract from the eyes, either.

HAIR

❃ The hairstyle here has been replaced with a necklace–cum–hair adornment. Part the hair into three sections, smoothing each section toward the back.

❃ Use bobby pins to secure the ends of the necklace onto the hair.

Takeaway tip: Beauty comes in all colors and from all cultures. Experiment with a new look inspired by a culture you admire.

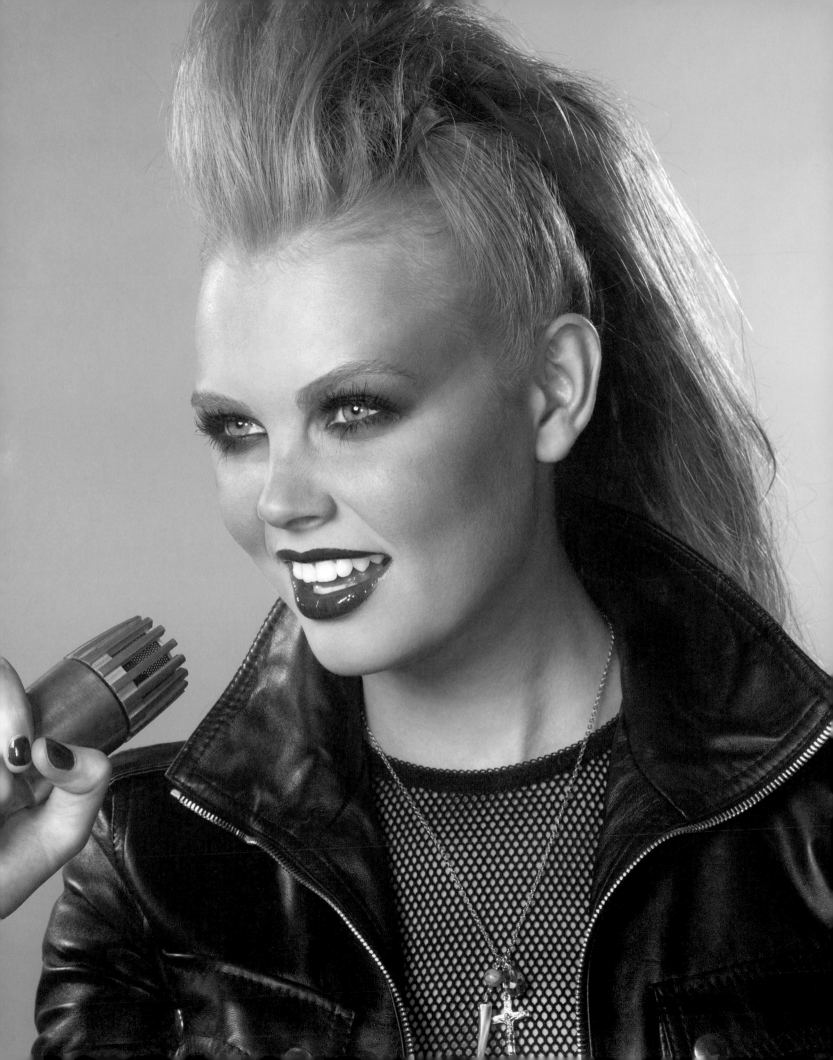

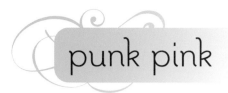

punk pink

This look is a rule-breaker: dark eyes with dark lips! It's a punk-inspired look that will make people look twice.

FACE

❋ Your skin needs to be immaculate in order to pull off such extreme makeup. Use a matte foundation to even and perfect skin tone and cover discoloration.

❋ Finish with a dusting of loose translucent powder to set the makeup.

CHEEKS

❋ Pick a strong, rose-toned blush. Apply to the apples of the cheeks. Blend up and back, making the blush appear with plenty of color.

EYES

❋ Use a pink-toned matte shadow in the crease, instead of the usual contour color. Exaggerate the contouring, extending it to the inner eye and out beyond the brow bone.

❋ Use a lighter-toned pink eye shadow along the brow bone and extend it down and past the outer edge of the eye. From there, extend a streak of pink all the way back to the hairline.

❋ With a sharpened black eyeliner pencil, draw along the entire top lash line. Extend the line outward beyond the eye in a medium-width, straight stroke.

❋ With the pencil, extend the line to the inner eye, exaggerating the inner eye point.

❋ Apply a strip of fake lashes to the top lash line.

❋ Apply mascara, and rock on!

LIPS

❋ Line the lips with a strong red lip-liner in a shade slightly darker than, but still complementary to, the lipstick shade. A dark lip color demands a very defined lip.

❋ Use a lip brush to apply a cream pink-red lip color over the lined lips. Blend well, but keep the strong lip line.

❋ The overall look is very youthful, so add a coat of gloss to keep the face fresh.

HAIR

❋ Separate the center section of the hair in one long, front-to-back mohawk strip.

❋ For the front section of the mohawk, tease and spray until you have a sizable pouf to play with.

❋ Tuck and smooth the ends of the front teased section into the hair directly behind the front section.

❋ Secure the side sections of hair along the top and back of the center strip with bobby pins. Secure the hair along the entire section, from front to back, anchoring each bobby pin into the base of the modified mohawk.

❋ Experiment with extensions. Each of these pink extensions has a clip on the base for ultra-easy use.

Takeaway tip: Everyone should try a rule-breaking, color-saturated look at least once.

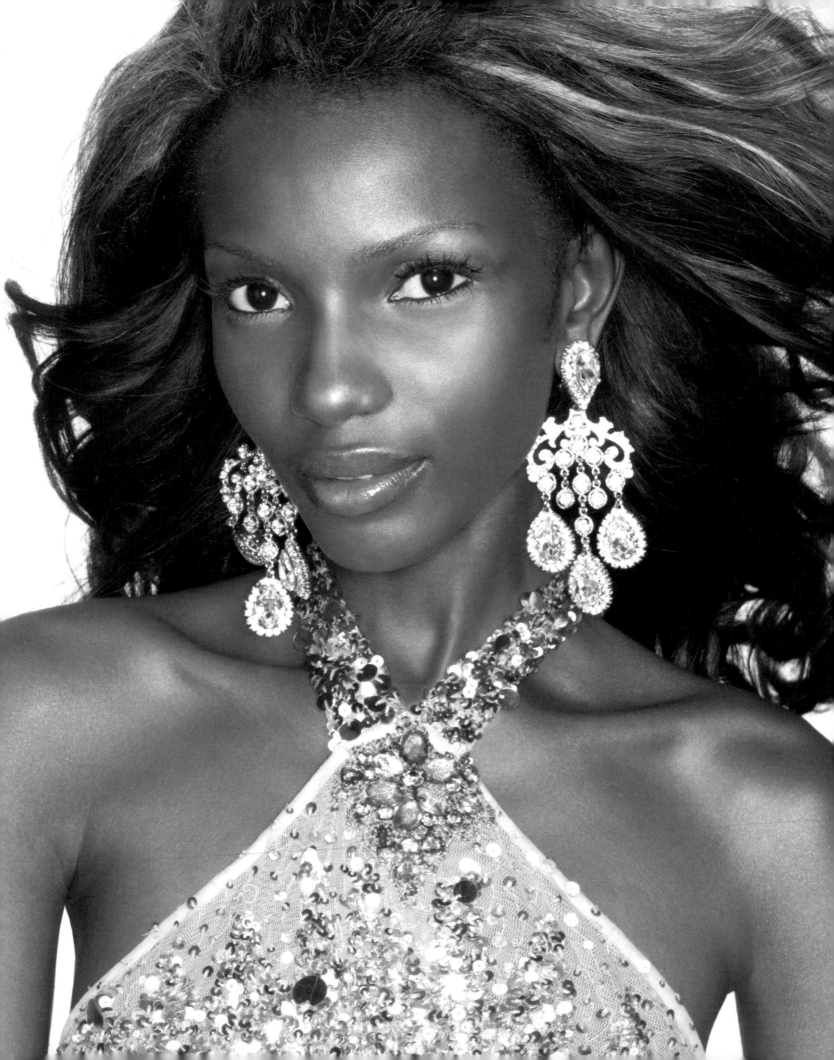

dangerous diva

Luminous, beautiful skin paired with smashing makeup takes you from the house party to the club.

FACE

❋ Smooth the skin with a mid-coverage foundation, which will even out dark areas and minimize blemishes. Sensual skin is key for a soft look, so don't overload on the foundation.

❋ Blend the foundation carefully with a damp sponge, to make the look still seem "breathable."

❋ To shape and contour the face, highlight the cheeks, the center of the nose, the temples, and the chin using an iridescent highlighting cream.

❋ Shade the hollows of the cheeks, jawline, and the side of the forehead with darker cream foundation or concealer, to make the face look slender.

CHEEKS

❋ A burst of bright pink blush on the apples of the cheeks gives a vivid flash of color. Use a cream blush and blend into the cheeks, leaving a seamless flush.

EYES

❋ Use light, high-glitter shadows for eyes that glow. Apply a highlighter to the inner eye and on the brow bone.

❋ Contour in a darker shade, but one that also is a shiny formula. Apply it under the brow bone and in the crease.

❋ On the lid, opt for a medium-tone, high-shimmer formula to create more definition.

❋ Use a black eyeliner pencil to line the lower rim.

❋ Apply gold eye shadow along the lower lash line.

❋ Skip the liner and go straight for the eyelash curler.

❋ Finish with mascara.

LIPS

❋ Full and lush lips need no liner. Simply apply a coating of golden pearlescent gloss.

HAIR

❋ Blondes come in all skin tones! Try a wig to experiment with a lighter, longer look.

❋ Be aware of the undertone of blonde you are picking. The consultant at the beauty supply store should be helpful in matching you with your best blonde shade, but I recommend you wear your makeup for this look to the store—or at least a toned-down version of it—so you can try different shades of blonde and make sure you buy the right one.

playful palettes

If trying a whole new look is too intimidating, opt to experiment with a different color palette.

1. BLUES

Blues are a cool, sophisticated color choice. Keep the lips simple with such strong eyes.

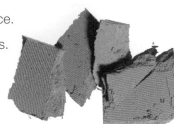

❋ **Cheeks:** deep-pink-toned blush on the cheeks

❋ **Eyes:** iridescent blue for the ball and crease of the lid, paired with a lighter blue as a highlighter

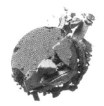 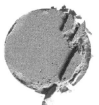

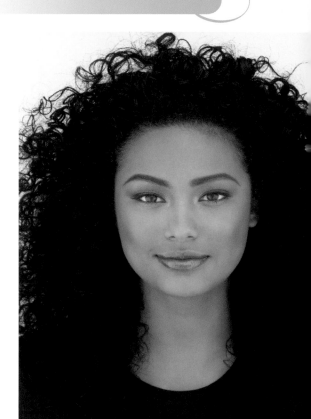

❋ **Lips:** sheer lip gloss in neutral shade

2. ORANGE

Orange is an unexpected selection. This look plays with orange and bronze.

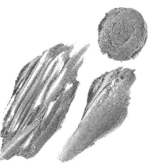

❋ **Cheeks:** citrine-like cream blush

❋ **Eyes:** mango-colored cream eye shadow

❋ **Lips:** bright tangerine gloss

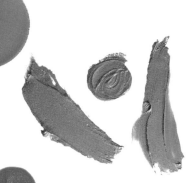

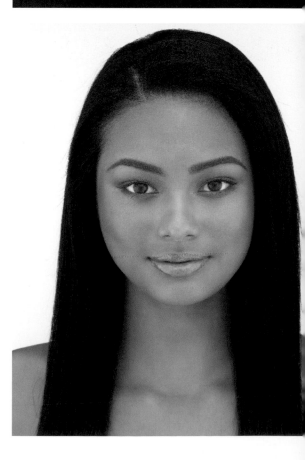

3. PINKS

Pink is not just for Barbie! A choice of warm, dusty pinks is an easy mix for everyday wear.

✳ **Cheeks:** earth-tone blush keeps the palette from looking too plasticky pink

✳ **Eyes:** gentle rosy lilac applied over the entire lid

✳ **Lips:** a soft pink gloss

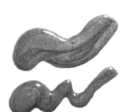

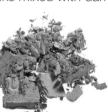

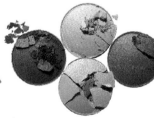

4. LAVENDER

You never knew pastel could be so bold.

✳ **Cheeks:** a purple-hued flush for the cachetes

✳ **Eyes:** deeper pinks mixed with darker lilacs create a colorful smoky eye

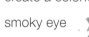

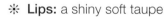

✳ **Lips:** a shiny soft taupe

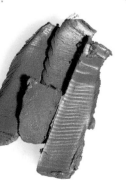

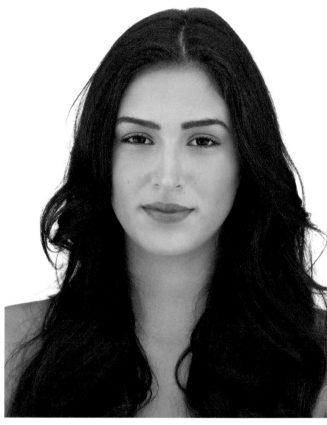

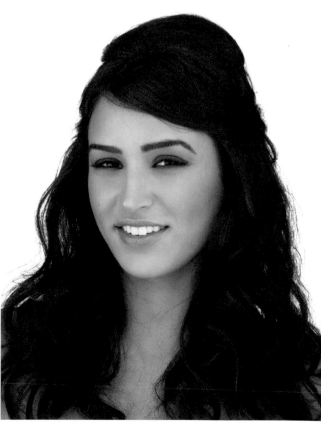

5. SILVERY PINKS

Pink packs a punch when silver is added to the mix.

* **Cheeks:** super-bright, very wearable

* **Eyes:** high-shimmer shadow creates a glossy eye

* **Lips:** a clear, pale pink glittery gloss

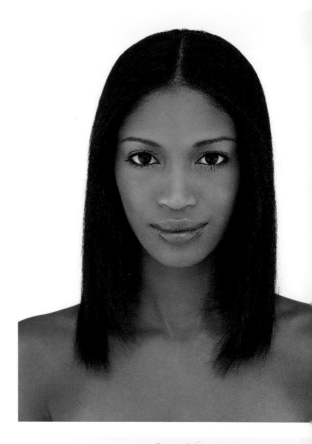

6. GUNMETAL SILVER

Gunmetal gray mixed with cool reds creates a combination that can handle dark eyes and dark lips.

* **Cheeks:** deep pink

* **Eyes:** saturated silver with a touch of metallic blue—sexy and dangerous

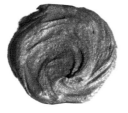

* **Lips:** deep red, almost burgundy in a sheer texture

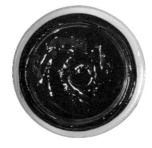

7. BROWN

Burnished, soft, and easy-to-apply neutrals prove that browns are never boring.

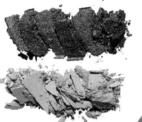

❋ **Cheeks:** golden blush

❋ **Eyes:** a dusty pink all-over lid color with a warm brown for contour

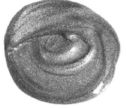

❋ **Lips:** peach gloss

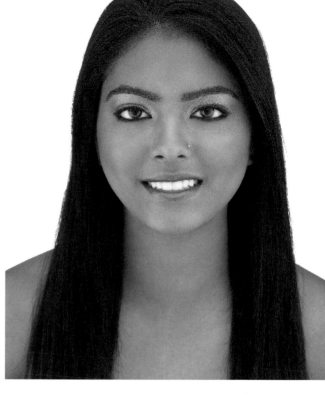

8. BRONZE

Radiating a honey glow, bronzers get bold for an evening look.

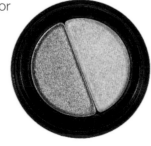

❋ **Cheeks:** liquid bronzer

❋ **Eyes:** burnished gold for highlighter, copper for lid color

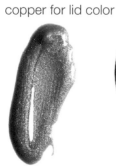

❋ **Lips:** shimmery brown

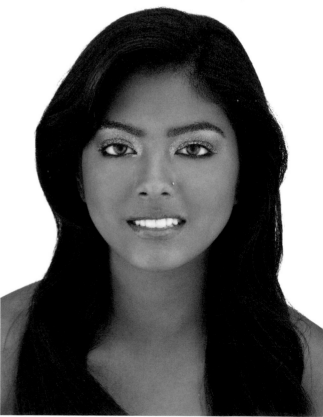

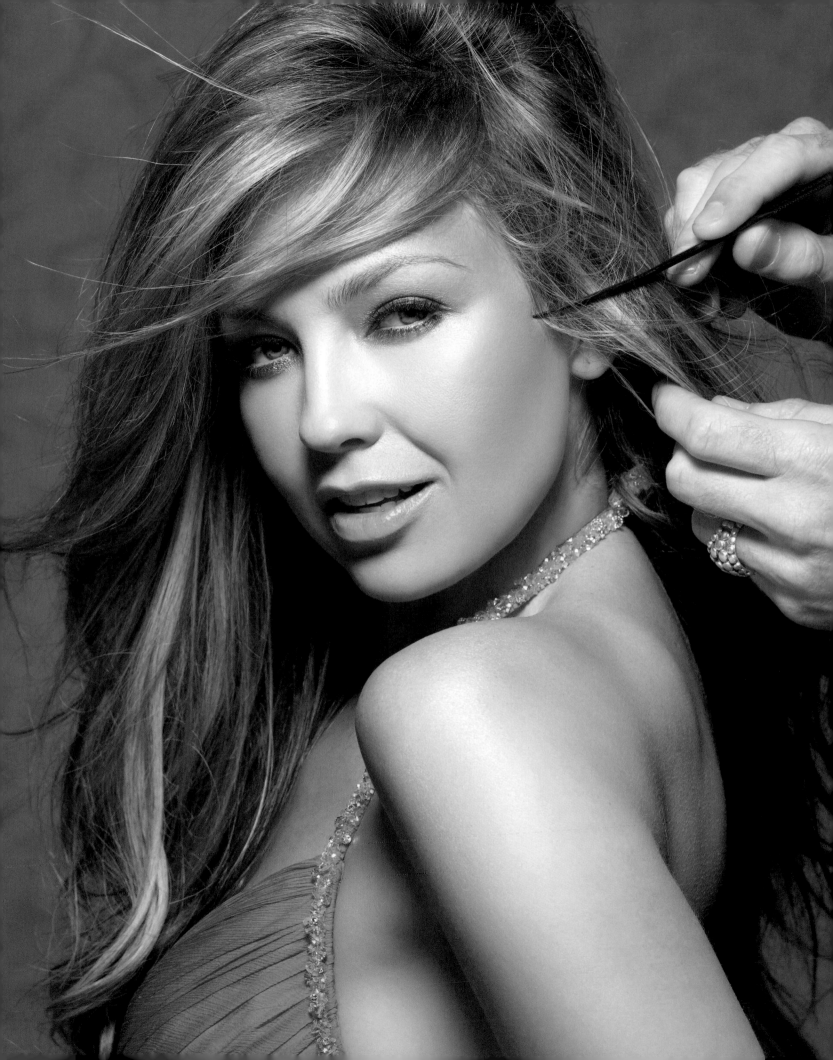

red-carpet ready

SPECIAL EVENTS PREP

Quinceañeras, bodas, and the red carpet—I've done them all, and I've learned as much from my mistakes as from my successes. It's hard to know if what looks cool in your bedroom will bomb in photographs or will just feel somehow wrong when all eyes are upon you. Before strutting down the red carpet, I've had my hair teased, colored, curled, straightened, and pinned into any number of different styles that were super-hip at the moment.

In this chapter I offer you foolproof tips and tricks to help you feel great about how you look on your special day, so you can concentrate on having fun. I'll teach you how to re-create five of my favorite red-carpet looks. I'll explain my best tips for taking a flattering photograph—it's taken me years of practice, but I've finally nailed it!

But first, let's discuss the age-old debate: traditional vs. trendy. It's a decision to consider carefully whenever you'll be going to a special event, especially when you want to be remembered as the star of the show.

traditional vs. trendy

Weddings and quinceañeras are moments when the more classic you look, the better. Girls celebrating their quince have more leeway—after all, when you are fourteen or fifteen, anything looks good on you! But in general, when you are thinking about the look you want for your special day, remember that you and your family will be looking at these pictures for years to come. Now that I am an adult, and I can look at things from a larger perspective, I see that it's best to opt for classic beauty, which will look timeless and stunning in photographs years from now.

Not that *I* actually did that. Out there on the World Wide Web for everyone to see and download are tons of pictures of me in my teens, when I thought less was less and that more was . . . fabulous! The heavy foundation, the matte red lips, the Aqua Net hair—I did it all. I looked very much the part of a teenager in the '80s. It's like someone let me loose at the department store beauty counter and I decided to try everything on my face at once, kind of like Boy George. In my quinceañera photos I am sporting a Mexican interpretation of a Duran Duran hairdo and—yes indeed—a sweatband à la Olivia Newton-John. I may have looked ridiculous, but I felt like I was the flyest girl in the room, and no one could tell me anything different. And at the end of the day, that is what I wish for every girl who is contemplating how she will do her makeup and hair on her quinceañera. Whatever you decide to do, you should end up feeling like you are the star!

For quinceañeras, the focus should be more on combining classic beauty with a modern twist. My personal preference is also that quince girls look their age, not like a thirty-five-year-old vamp. The goal should be a playful, fun, and fresh look, nothing too sexy. There is plenty of time to look sexy. Now is the time to have fun. For makeup, choose eye shadows with a little glitter or shimmer. Use beautiful, flirty fake eyelashes on the outer sections of the lash line. Stay away from dark or smoky eyes. Make your cheeks rosy pink. Lorac has a great phosphorescent pink that looks amazing when applied. Try a plumping lip gloss for to-the-max shine and shape. For your hair, choose a style that is fresh. You are going to dance, sweat, laugh, kiss all your friends and loved ones, and be the center of attention. The focus should be on having fun. That is something I *did* do right with my quinceañera look: I had fun. I had my costurera knock off a Dior dress from an ad I found in *Vogue*. At that time, Molly Ringwald was la maxima para mi—the top style icon. I made my hair Cyndi Lauper–ish, with my satin sweatband replacing the tiara. That was my way of giving my look a modern twist.

On December 2, 2000, I got married in Saint Patrick's Cathedral in New York City. Man, *that* was a big event. There were more than five hundred invited guests, including Robert De Niro, Bruce Springsteen, Gloria Estefan, Jennifer Lopez, Michael Jackson, and of course my crazy, always fun Mexican friends. About ten thousand of my loyal fans had also traveled to New York to be with me on my special day. Half of Fifth Avenue was closed down. I definitely needed to look good! For my wedding, I chose Disney's Cinderella as inspiration for my hair, makeup, and dress. My eyes were lined with dark brown liner that was applied to look catlike and coquettish. I even made my brows stronger with pencil, just like Cinderella's. Since my eyes were the focal

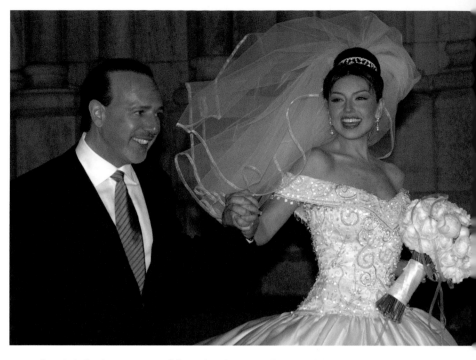

point, I did my lips in a neutral color. I applied creamy lipstick for long, wearable color. I wanted to avoid gloss, which I worried might stick to my veil or might not last beyond the priest's "You may kiss the bride." My hair was also adapted from the Disney movie: a modernized beehive up-do with eye-framing bangs. Instead of the black headband that Cinderella wears, I wore a tiara with diamonds.

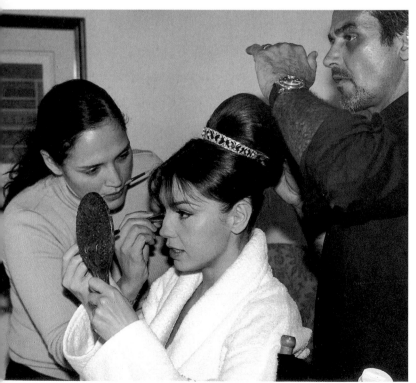

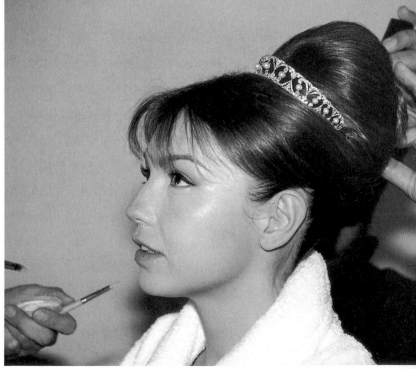

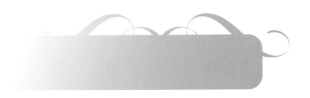

paparazzi perfect

The red carpet is my runway. I play around with different styles and different looks depending on my dress and mood. No matter what I wear, how I do my hair, or what makeup I choose, I always want to feel like myself—it could be the rebel, the siren, or the girl next door in me, but it's still me.

Yes, for some of these red-carpet events, I had the help of a professional glam squad—a stylist, makeup artist, and hairstylist—to help me create these looks, but I've kept the how-tos here as simple as possible, so you can try them on your own.

greek goddess

I was channeling Aphrodite, goddess of love, with this look. I wore this glorious gown to the 2005 Billboard Latin Music Awards.

MAKEUP The peachy lips are the focus of the face. I used a lip-liner to give my lips definition, then a sheer color on top. I applied a peachy-bronze blusher to the apples of my cheeks for a pop of color. My eye makeup was also in the bronze color family. I used a highlighter on the brow bone to open up my eye. A contour shadow in the crease gave me added definition and depth, so my eyes would not be washed out in the glare of the photographers' flashes. On the ball of my eyelid, I applied a golden shimmor to draw light to my eyes. Eyeliner on the top outer third of my lash line made my eyes appear bigger, and a generous application of mascara finished the look.

HAIR First, my hair was blown out to a sleek and shiny smoothness. The top center section was back-combed for height, then smoothed over to keep the height but create a clean look, then secured at the crown with bobby pins neatly tucked in. The rest of my hair was pulled back into a sleek ponytail secured at the nape of my neck. A shine serum was smoothed onto my ponytail, so I would avoid flyaways.

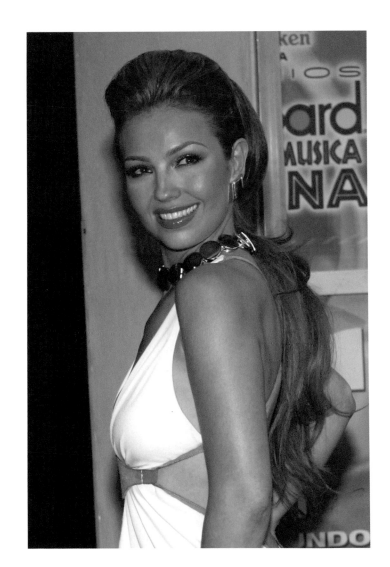

sleek and simple

One of the biggest beauty risks to take is to pull the hair back completely, with no bangs or lingering wisps to frame the face. There's nothing to hide behind—especially when paired with the spare, spaghetti-strap neckline of a dress like this one. That is exactly why I tried it and exactly why it is one of my favorite red-carpet looks. I wore it to the 2003 Latin Grammys.

MAKEUP The red dress was a strong color statement, so I kept my makeup simple and flattering. My brows were strong. My makeup was in neutral tones, but I applied toned blusher to the apples of my cheeks. I applied some brown contour in the crease of my eyes, some soft gray eye shadow on my lids, and used dark brown eyeliner along the top lashes. I applied false eyelashes, too, followed by mascara.

HAIR My hair was blown out straight. It was then pulled off my face, the sides and top slicked with gel, and secured in the back with an elastic. A lock from the ponytail was wrapped around the elastic. The end was secured under the ponytail with hidden bobby pins. The ponytail was curled with a curling iron for some movement

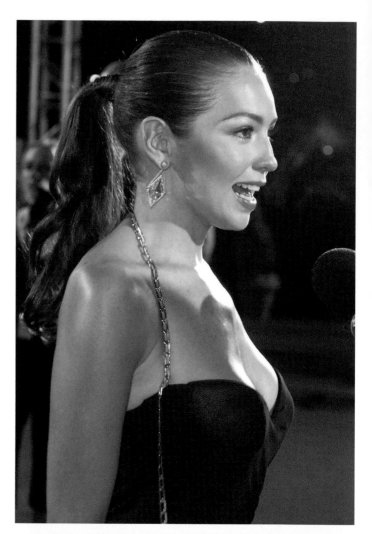

indian princess

I loved the color and drama of this sari-inspired dress. I wore it to the 2002 Latin Grammys. It made me feel regal and unique.

MAKEUP My eyes had the traditional kohl that Indian women apply for ultra-smoky eyes. I applied liquid liner along my top lash line and extended it up. I wore a coral lip color.

HAIR Since the dress and the makeup were so dramatic, I kept my hair as simple as possible. I flat-ironed; it was then pulled back into a ponytail at the nape of my neck. Serum gave my strands a glossy, smooth finish.

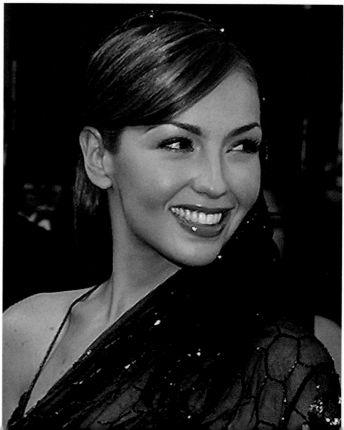

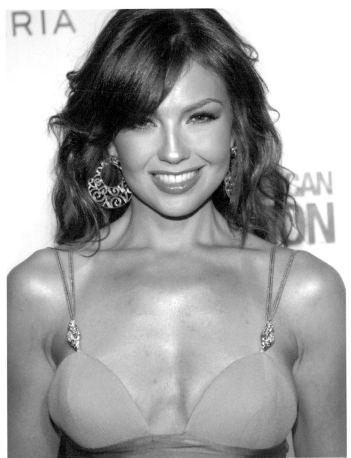

tangerine dream

This bright, electric-coral dress paired with soft, loose hair is the look I chose for the 2005 Fashion Rocks show.

MAKEUP The vivid orange of the dress demanded pretty, subtle makeup in a bronzed, burnished color family. I used a pinkish peach on my cheeks and added bronzer. After lining my lips with a neutral, orange-toned pencil, I applied a sparkly tangerine gloss to shine and shape.

HAIR Curvaceous waves were a wonderful complement to this body-hugging gown. Large hot rollers gave my waves body and movement and shaped them around my face with a deep side part and side-swept bangs. A light coating of hair spray helped ensure that my waves would hold.

luxe look

Since I was going to the Victoria's Secret Fashion Show in 2005, I thought the smoldering, sex-kitten look was appropriate.

MAKEUP Dark, catlike eyes and light lips created this retro style. I kept the eye shadow simple and in neutral tones. I used a simple shimmery base color with a warm contour shade in the crease. I applied liquid liner to the top lash line, extending the end outward and upward slightly beyond my eye. False eyelashes topped with black mascara, especially on the outer lashes, completed my eye makeup. I used a dusty-rose blush on my cheeks. I lined my lips with skin-colored liner and topped it off with a soft golden gloss.

HAIR My hair was styled to look like tousled, sexy, bed-head hair, similar to the ultra-feminine styles of the 1950s. The top section of hair was teased to give it height, then smoothed over with a brush and secured at the crown with bobby pins. The back and sides were curled with a large-barrel curling iron to create loose, sensual curls. And finally, I gently separated and finger-combed my soft curls. This is one of my favorite hairdos because my face is so round, the height at the top is slimming.

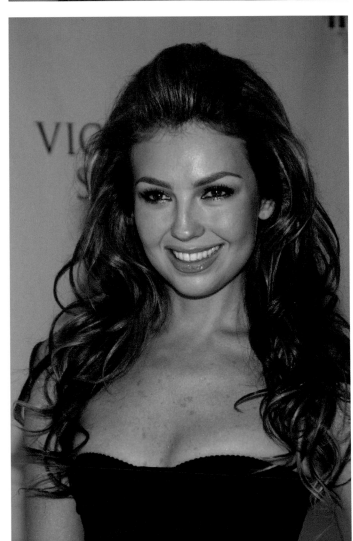

posing without being a poser

Look at the two photos here. In one, I have what I call my "Thalia face," as in the Thalia face that the public has come to know. In the second, which shows the right side of my face, my face looks much rounder—you see the baby fat. At a three-quarter angle, my left side is far more defined and simply looks better on film. Unfortunately, I found this out the hard way, with my chubby side staring back at me in all my early paparazzi moments. Hopefully, you won't suffer the same public exposure!

No one's face is completely symmetrical. So when you have a big event coming up—especially if you're paying a photographer to capture memories that you will look back on for years—there is no shame in posing in front of the mirror until you find your best angle. With digital cameras, it's even easier to check yourself out. The camera will you tell you truths—immediately!—that even your closest friends may not. For that reason, I'd advise you to take your digital camera with you when you have your trial makeup applied, and when you are trying to decide on the hairstyle to wear with your dress, tiara, or veil. The digital pics will give you a sense of what works in terms of your makeup and what does not; which features the flash washes out and which features look just right. Here are some other pointers for taking a fabulous photograph:

❊ Strong opaque colors in the red and blue family can look harsh on film. Instead of red lipstick, opt for berry or wine tones. On the eyes, apply dark navy or sheer muted blues. Steer clear of overly bright matte blues and cool-toned harsh reds—unless you are expert at their application.

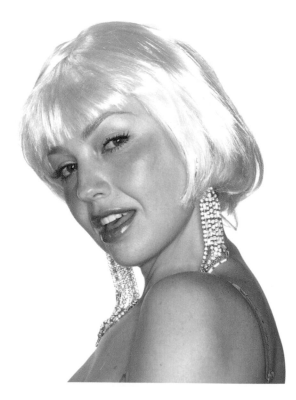
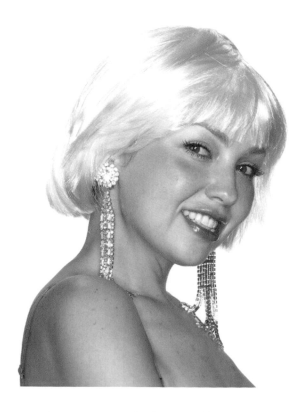

❋ Apply powder in the A-shape we talked about in the "Laying a Great Foundation" chapter: it will eliminate the bad shine while still allowing your skin to look fresh and dewy for the camera.

❋ Practice your smile. A huge grin that spreads across your face a mile wide is a spontaneous expression of joy and happiness. But, in photographs, especially posed ones, such a beaming expression can squint up your eyes, making you look a little goofy. Snap some pictures of yourself smiling to get a sense of what your best smile is in a photograph. If you are really good at it, you can have a few practiced smiles that you like: one with teeth, one with no teeth, a bright smile, a subtle smile, etc.

❋ Eliminate that double chin! Remember how E.T. could stretch his head out and make his neck super-long? That's what you are going to do. Keep your shoulders back, hold your tongue to the roof of your mouth— an instant neck lift without going under the knife!—and slightly stretch your face out and away from your chest. Your face will look sleek and slender.

❋ Try not to be the victim of a bad photographer. Make sure that his or her lens is placed at your face level or higher. The ideal position is to have the lens looking down at you, which automatically takes pounds off your face, neck, and shoulders. The opposite—when you are looking down at the camera—will add years, wrinkles, and poundage, making you look like a new breed of shar-pei.

❋ You know how everyone makes fun of the beauty-queen stance? Let me tell you something, cariño: there is a reason those girls stand the way they do. And the reason is that one can drop twelve pounds quickly— at least in a photograph—if she stands with her body at a three-quarter angle to the camera, places one foot slightly in front of the other, and sucks in la panza.

❋ Keep your arms loose but at your side. Crossing them in front of you makes your shoulders look broad.

❋ Wearing strapless dress? For a picture, place your hands on your hips, throw the tops of your shoulders forward, and that little underarm bulge will disappear faster than a plastic surgeon can wave a liposuction canula at it.

❋ If you're taking a group picture, try to stand slightly behind the other people in the photograph. Drape your arm behind the back of the person standing next to you, but not over his or her shoulder or behind the neck. Drape your arm around his or her waist or lower back. Visually, you will look smaller. Let the beauty queens keep the close-fingered wave. You don't need to do that. Feeling a bit bloated instead of svelte and sexy? During the inevitable group picture, put one leg behind the person beside you. That way you are three-quarters covered from the unforgiving, fat-adding camera lens.

❋ Stand up straight! No hunched shoulders!

Here's what I always carry in my evening clutch:

Eyelash glue • Powder compact • Gloss • Makeup brush with one application of bronzer wrapped in tissue • Breath mints (remember all that kissing—don't kill your friends with a whiff of bad breath!)

ready for your close-up, cariño?

I am a lighting control freak. It's kind of inevitable when your job is to look at your face every day and you start to analyze what makes you look your best. Even when I am going into a conference room for a business meeting, or sitting down in a restaurant, I am aware of where to sit to get the "power" lighting. You can't live your life obsessing about lighting, but at least you can learn from my years of surviving in this business. Knowing what looks best can help you relax in front of the camera.

❋ Photographers' lights tend to pick up and exaggerate shine. Go very lightly with highlighters and use a matte formula foundation on your nose, forehead, and chin—the areas that tend to get shiny— especially if you will be nervous that day. Keep blotting papers handy for quick touch-ups before you go in front of the camera.

❋ I try to avoid the kind of overhead lighting that bears straight down. It makes everyone look bad. This type of lighting creates shadows in the crease of the mouth and in the hollows of your eyes.

❋ Can't avoid that lighting? Create your own Marilyn Monroe moment (she was an absolute expert at how to best position herself to look amazing in every picture) and tilt your face slightly upward. This will bathe your face in the overhead light, eliminating the shadows.

❋ If you are in a well-lit room with natural light streaming in from the windows, sit facing the windows. This will give you a better glow than if a lighting tech had done it as you sat for a portrait with a professional photographer.

■ CELEB SECRET REVEALED! ■

Before applying makeup on me for a big event, my makeup artist often starts with a face mask to soothe and prepare my skin. The face mask isn't greasy or heavy. It hydrates and softens my skin, making it feel tingly and supple. Use a mask you've tried before so you don't, God forbid, break out in a rash before your big day. My makeup artist also recommends facial massage to help eliminate puffiness. This mini facial massage is so easy, you can even do it on yourself. It has the added bonus of relaxing you—always a nice thing on a day that will inevitably be fraught with frazzled nerves.

Using your ring finger, gently apply pressure to center of your chin. Make tiny circles as you go back along your jawline to the tip of your earlobe.

Start again at the center right beneath your bottom lip. Again, move your ring finger in tiny circular movements out toward the middle of the edge of your ear.

Start again at the center right above your upper lip. Again, move your ring finger in tiny circular movements outward and upward toward your temple.

Finish by placing your ring fingers in the middle of your forehead, making tiny circles outward until you reach the temples.

This will help stimulate blood flow and ease puffiness in your face.

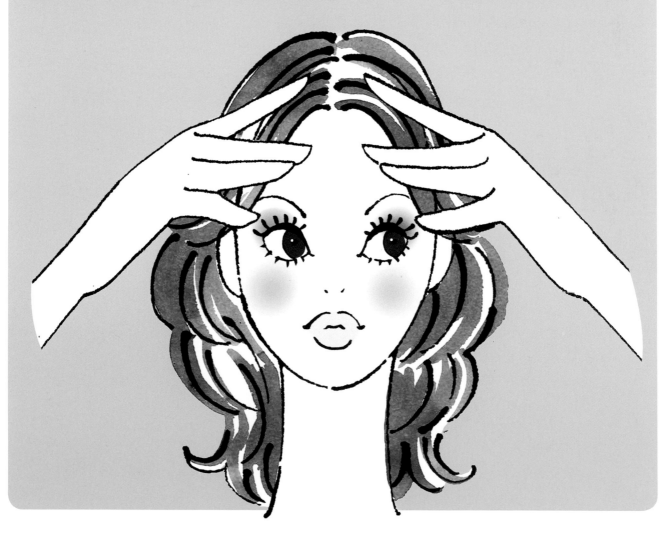

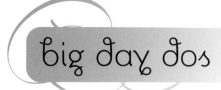

big day dos

You can't control everything on your big day: the weather, your primo Chewy's corny jokes, the DJ wandering from your playlist. But the little beauty details? Totally doable!

❈ Too much foundation or powder will look heavy or like a white mask in photographs when a flash is used. Apply loose powder sparingly and try to dry the T-zone with blotting sheets instead of piling on more powder. You also can simply dab at your face with a tissue. It will lift some of the oil without removing any makeup.

❈ Highlighters are tricky when it comes to photography, so use them sparingly. Wearing too much highlighter will make your skin look oily.

❈ Prevent eyeliner from running by applying similar-colored eye shadow over the eyeliner with a stiff-bristled eye brush immediately after you've lined your eye. This is to set eyeliner, as you similarly set your face using loose powder after you have applied your face makeup.

❈ Use waterproof mascara and eyeliner! These won't budge in the case of either tears of joy or panicked tears of "What am I doing?!"

❈ If you'll be putting your hair in an up-do, make sure you have a trial run with your hairstylist. If you wait until the big day, you run the risk of making your up-do too tight! I have had my share of headaches because of hair that was pinned back too tightly. You might look good, but you'll feel like hell.

big day don'ts

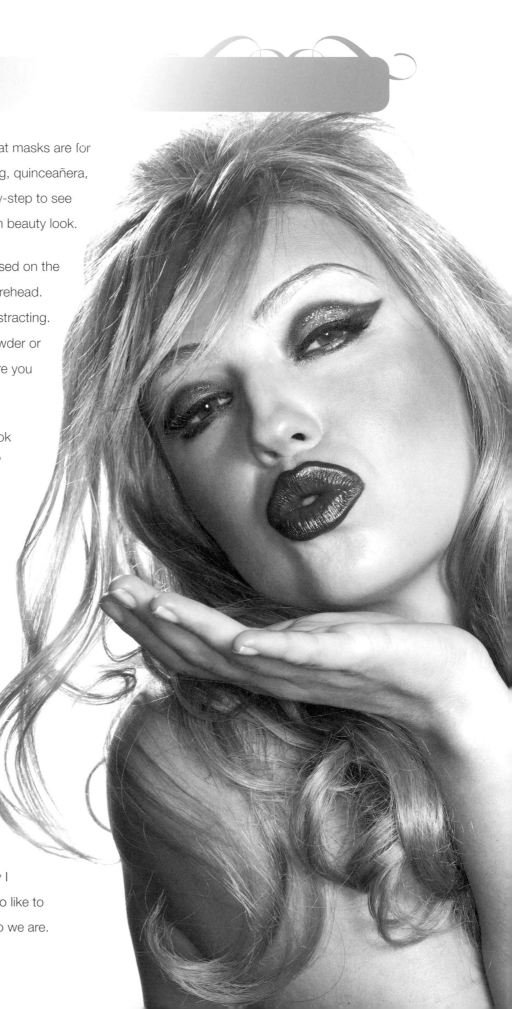

Holy guacamole! Somebody tell this chick that masks are for lucha libre fighters, not for going to a wedding, quinceañera, or out to a club! Let's go through this step-by-step to see what not to do for your next special-occasion beauty look.

BROWS Eyebrow pencils are meant to be used on the natural brow, not two inches above on the forehead. Ultra-thin penciled-in brows are aging and distracting. If you have seriously sparse brows, apply powder or pencil where your brows should be, not where you would like them to be.

EYE SHADOW You will never read in my book some random rule like "no blue eye shadow," because I've shown you how to make blue look beautiful. But this is a lesson in blue eye shadow gone wrong. Too much, too harsh, too bright.

LIP-LINER This chick obviously mistook her eyeliner for a lip-liner. In case there is any confusion, let me be clear: dark lip-liner with a lighter lip color is a don't. This started as a cool makeup technique in the hands of top makeup artists. It has morphed into a nightmare beauty don't that won't die.

HAIR I call this color tono cucaracha, or cockroach colored. Yellowish brassy blonds are evidence of a dye job gone bad. In theory I encourage and enjoy experimenting, but I also like to enhance, not change, what we have and who we are.

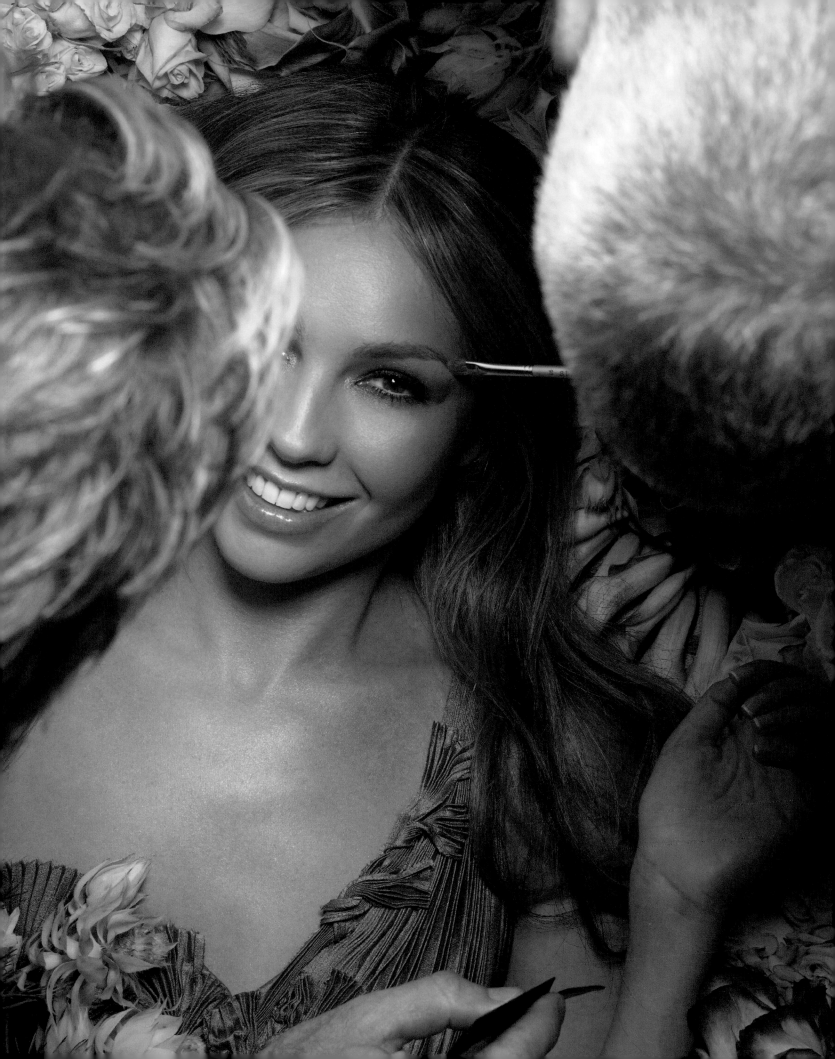

makeovers
REAL WOMEN, REAL CHANGES

For me, this isn't just a beauty book. It's a very personal expression of my private philosophies, ideas, and tips—a celebration of what it means to be beautiful inside and out. It's about loving what you look like before you put any makeup on, and then learning to have fun with your look and play with makeup and hair to accentuate the best version of yourself.

We all need a village of positive people to support us in feeling our best—that's why I wanted to include the people in my life who have been key to my own well-being, physically and emotionally. This chapter was a chance for me to honor the women who have been there for me for so long, teaching me so many lessons. To thank them, we gave them each a fabulous new look. Their makeovers represent beauty at every age. I hope you can steal the tips we gave them for yourself!

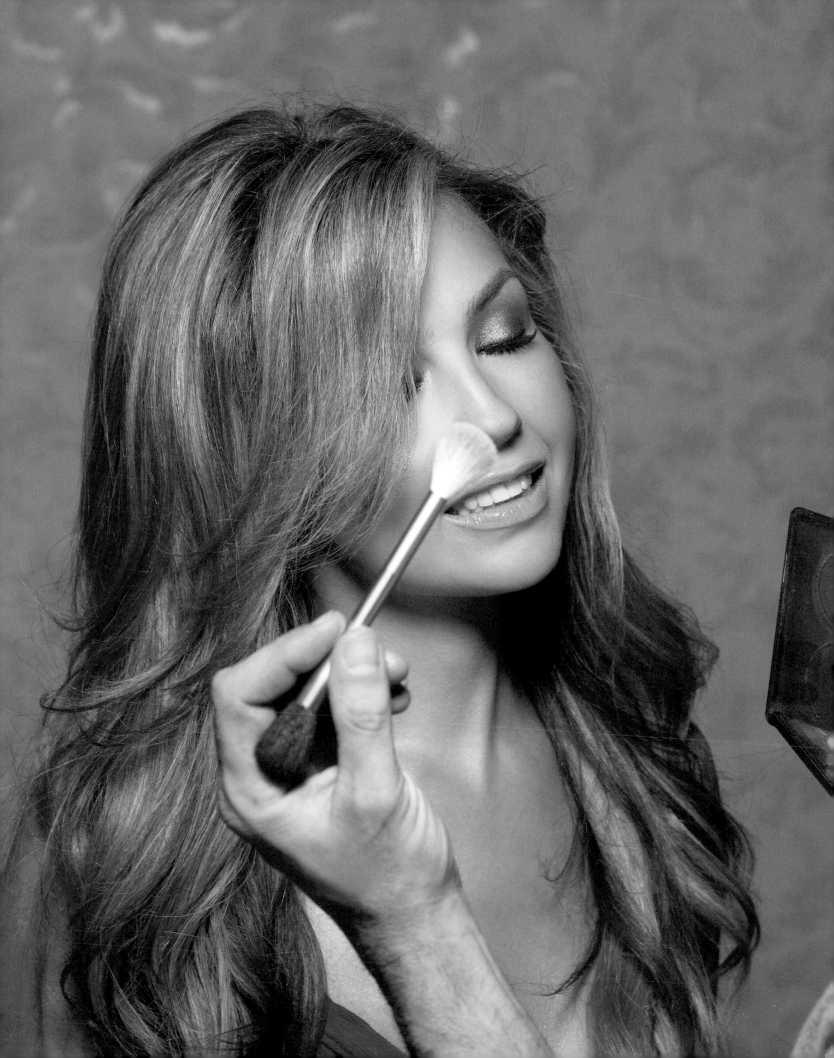

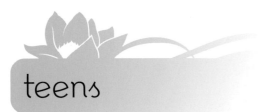

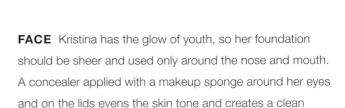

teens

kristina

Young women like Kristina, a student, continue to inspire and amaze me—proud of who they are and where they have come from, bursting with the beauty, energy, and dreams of young Latinas. I met Kristina through a woman who helped me with this book. After working together for so many hours, I told her I needed a teen for this section, and she told me about her niece Kristina. When I heard about Kristina's interest in fashion, her love of Indian movies, and how close she is to her family, I knew that she would be great for this book. Kristina's look is beautiful, playful, and international. I wanted her makeover to reflect the different cultures and sense of playfulness and adventure that influence her personal style.

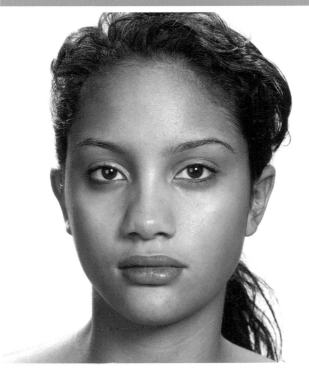

BEFORE A beautiful, fresh, clean face with big eyes just waiting to be noticed.

FACE Kristina has the glow of youth, so her foundation should be sheer and used only around the nose and mouth. A concealer applied with a makeup sponge around her eyes and on the lids evens the skin tone and creates a clean canvas.

CHEEKS Pink cream blush on the apples of her cheeks gives Kristina a glowing-from-within look and keeps a dewy texture to her skin.

EYES We used an eye-shadow brush to apply a pink eye shadow with minimal glitter particles. A green liquid eyeliner along the top lash line gives a pop of color. Light pink eye shadow on the inner corner and a squeeze of the eyelash curler and a generous sweep of black mascara on the top and bottom lashes. We tweezed her brows into a generous, clean shape.

LIPS A girl is nothing without her gloss, honey. A generous swipe of sugary pink sparkle gives a pop of color while keeping the entire look very youthful.

HAIR If you have Kristina's naturally curly hair, you know it is most beautiful when it is left loose and flowing. We allowed Kristina's hair to air-dry, then gently sprayed the ends and used gel to freshen and define the curls.

AFTER ¡Coqueta! We applied simple shimmery makeup to emphasize Kristina's best features without making her look older than she really is.

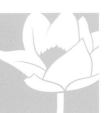

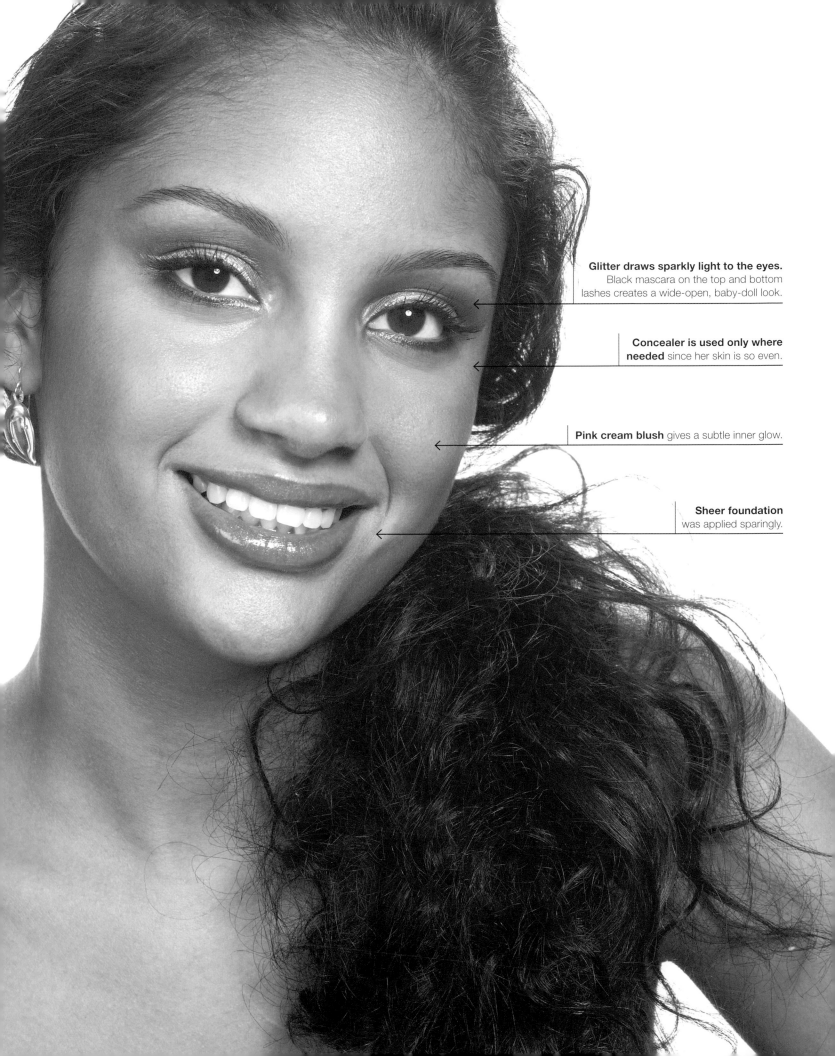

Glitter draws sparkly light to the eyes. Black mascara on the top and bottom lashes creates a wide-open, baby-doll look.

Concealer is used only where needed since her skin is so even.

Pink cream blush gives a subtle inner glow.

Sheer foundation was applied sparingly.

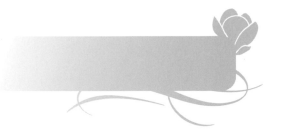

twenties

yudelka

Delka, a stay-at-home mom, is a lovely friend who I always run into in the far-flung corners of the world: Capri, St. Tropez, Cannes. We meet up in these random places and have the time of our lives. I call Delka an urban jet-setter, because she always remains close to her family and her roots while still traveling and enjoying the good life. She was happy to be a part of this project and even brought her bebíta to the set so we could all enjoy it together. With her sultry, magnetic looks, Delka is a true beauty.

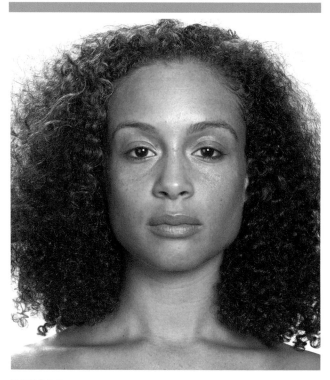

BEFORE A beautiful, natural girl with perfect skin and striking features.

FACE Delka's skin is even-toned, with tiny pores and minimal discoloration. (¡Suertudota!) We prepared her skin with a light hydrating cream and used foundation and concealer sparingly.

CHEEKS A little bronzer gives a flush of color to Delka's face, but we used it lightly, so that her cheeks and skin would not look washed out in comparison to her eyes.

EYES This eye look is smoky and steamy. We prepped Delka's eye area with eye cream and a light-reflecting concealer, and we used an eye-shadow brush to apply a shimmery golden color to her lids as a base. We applied it on the ball of the eye and extended the color up into the brow bone.

Starting along the lash line, we applied a matte dark-gray eye shadow along the top and bottom of her eyes, building layer by layer. The inner rim was lined with black pencil. We used individual clumps of false eyelashes and applied them to the outer lash line. We nestled each clump as close to the lash line as possible, interspersing them with Delka's own lashes.

We followed with a squeeze from the eyelash curler to give the eyes a great lift, then applied black mascara as the finishing step. And we didn't neglect the brows! After shaping and grooming them with tweezers and a brow brush, we used eyebrow powder to fill in any sparse areas and sealed the brows with clear brow gel.

LIPS Going for a dark lip look here would have been overkill for Delka. We opted to keep her lips smooth, glossy, and glowing with a peachy-golden-toned gloss.

HAIR If you have hair like Delka's, pump up those curls, muchacha! This creates a glorious, golden-hued halo for the face. We used a gel and a light spray on Delka's dry hair to scrunch and build the curls for extra height and body around the face.

AFTER A hot mama, ready to board the yacht in the south of France with a glass of champagne in one hand and her daughter in the other.

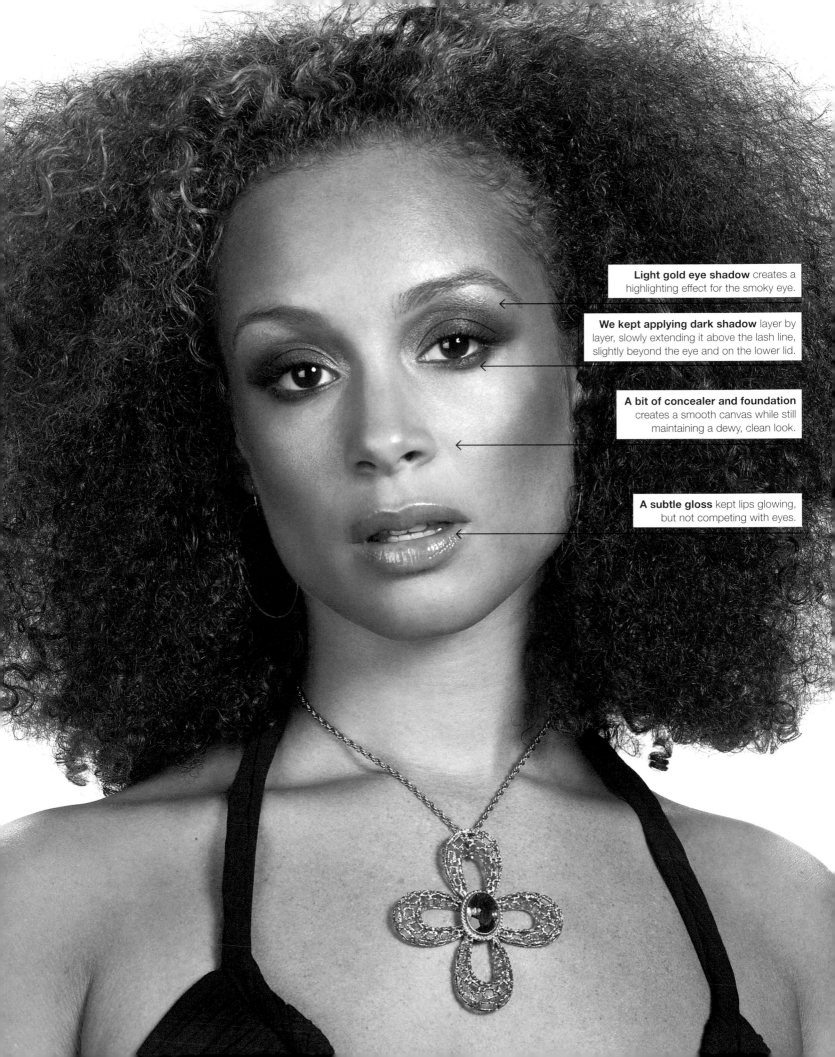

Light gold eye shadow creates a highlighting effect for the smoky eye.

We kept applying dark shadow layer by layer, slowly extending it above the lash line, slightly beyond the eye and on the lower lid.

A bit of concealer and foundation creates a smooth canvas while still maintaining a dewy, clean look.

A subtle gloss kept lips glowing, but not competing with eyes.

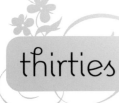

thirties

peggy

Peggy teaches me about the importance of the balance between soul and body, spirit and mind. She is an incredible and talented acupuncturist who not only helps me to reenergize but also helps me release stress and anxiety. I love her acupuncture facials, in which she uses needles around the face to promote healthy skin. Peggy is always on the run, doing work for so many celebrities. She is so in demand for her talents and gifts that I wanted her to slow down for a minute and do something for herself. This was her chance to have fun.

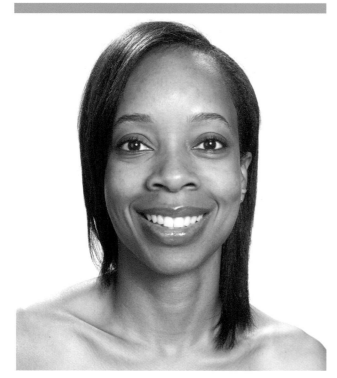

BEFORE Sculpture-worthy cheekbones are in there, I know they are.

FACE We applied a liquid foundation with a dampened sponge to create a matte, even-toned canvas. We used pointillism—the secret makeup-artist trick I shared with you in the chapter "Laying a Great Foundation"—to banish brown spots, cover blemishes, and minimize bumps.

CHEEKS We used a darker contour in the hollows of Peggy's cheeks, along her jawline, and along the sides of her nose to shape her face. Next we placed a highlighter directly above the apples of her cheeks, down the center of her nose, and on her chin to brighten the areas we wanted to accentuate, and blended vigorously and smoothly. This technique brought out the planes in her beautiful face. Finally, a spot of blush in a warm red hue gave her a healthy flush.

EYES We started with a light brown for the ball of the eye and as a base of color for her entire lid. A darker brown shadow in the crease and extended slightly upward and outward emphasizes the almond shape. We applied light, pearlescent highlighter in a pinkish hue to her brow bone.

LIPS A bold red takes anybody's look to a whole new level of excitement. We primed Peggy's supple exfoliated lips with a layer of waxy balm, then lined them with a nude-tone lip-liner to create a defined lip line. We used the liner to fill in her lips as well, for an even canvas for the lip color. Finally, we placed a dot of red gloss in the lower, fuller area of the lips to highlight that sexy, sensual lower lip.

HAIR We wanted a total and playful change, so we used extensions in a shade lighter than her natural color. You also can secure extensions with extensions glue, which comes out when you shampoo your hair. Anything more complicated than that, and I'd suggest you do what Peggy did: put yourself in the hands of a professional stylist.

AFTER Peggy reminds me of Donna Summer with fierce makeup and bold, red lips.

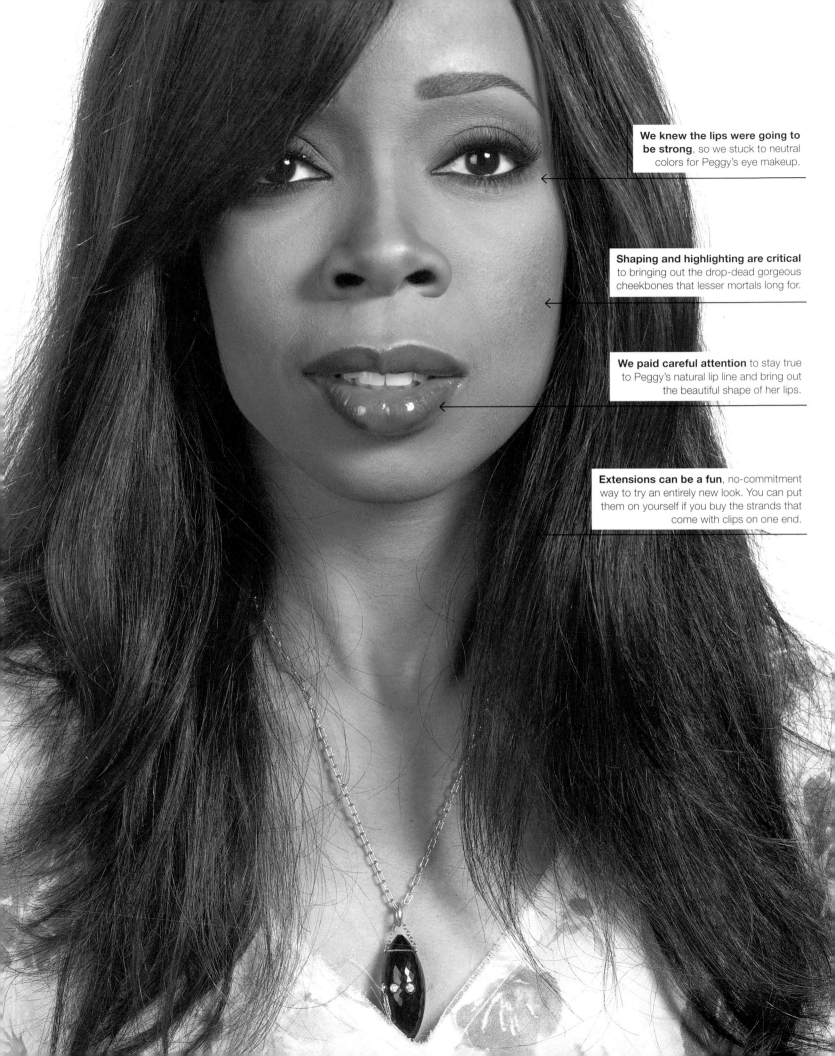

We knew the lips were going to be strong, so we stuck to neutral colors for Peggy's eye makeup.

Shaping and highlighting are critical to bringing out the drop-dead gorgeous cheekbones that lesser mortals long for.

We paid careful attention to stay true to Peggy's natural lip line and bring out the beautiful shape of her lips.

Extensions can be a fun, no-commitment way to try an entirely new look. You can put them on yourself if you buy the strands that come with clips on one end.

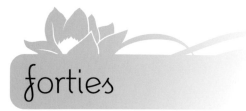

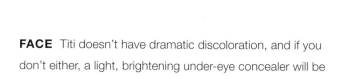

forties

ernestina

My sister Titi, a writer, is the founder of the optimists' club. She can transform any bad experience into a beneficial and life-affirming lesson. I believe she was put on this earth to teach love and commitment. And as for her beauty, she not only looks incredible for being in her forties, she also is the picture of how beauty emanates from the inside out. Titi projects positive energy. People are drawn to her. When you have such beauty inside, such a big heart, it comes out and makes you look ¡in-cre-í-ble!

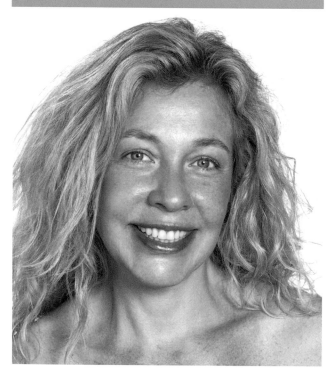

BEFORE You see it even without a hint of makeup on her face: my sister's eyes and her smile are her best features.

FACE Titi doesn't have dramatic discoloration, and if you don't either, a light, brightening under-eye concealer will be all you need to prepare your face.

CHEEKS We applied a pop of pink-hued powder blush on the apples to give Titi a nice flush of color and accentuate her beautiful cheeks and prominent cheekbones.

EYES Titi's smoky eye makeup here is a sophisticated, toned-down version of Delka's eye makeup. We used a deep copper, rather than the gray we used with Delka, to highlight the brilliant blue of Titi's eyes, making them the focus of her face. We applied a pearlescent pink as a base and used an eye-shadow brush to blend the color up toward her brow bone. With a smaller eye-shadow brush we applied a bronzed shadow along her upper and lower lash lines. On the lid, we extended the shadow up and blended it into the crease of her eye.

LIPS A rich berry-hued gloss complements Titi's rose-colored cheeks without competing with her dramatic eyes.

HAIR Titi's natural hair is wavy to curly. A sleek 'do goes well with this sexy look, so if your hair texture is like Titi's, start with wet hair and apply a straightening balm to protect the hair from the heat (and ensure a no-frizz finish), then blow your locks straight with a hair dryer, section by section, using a round large-barrel brush. A few drops of smoothing serum seal the cuticle and amp up the shine factor.

AFTER With this va-va-voom, ultra-glam look, she's ready to walk the red carpet, a trail of photographers behind her.

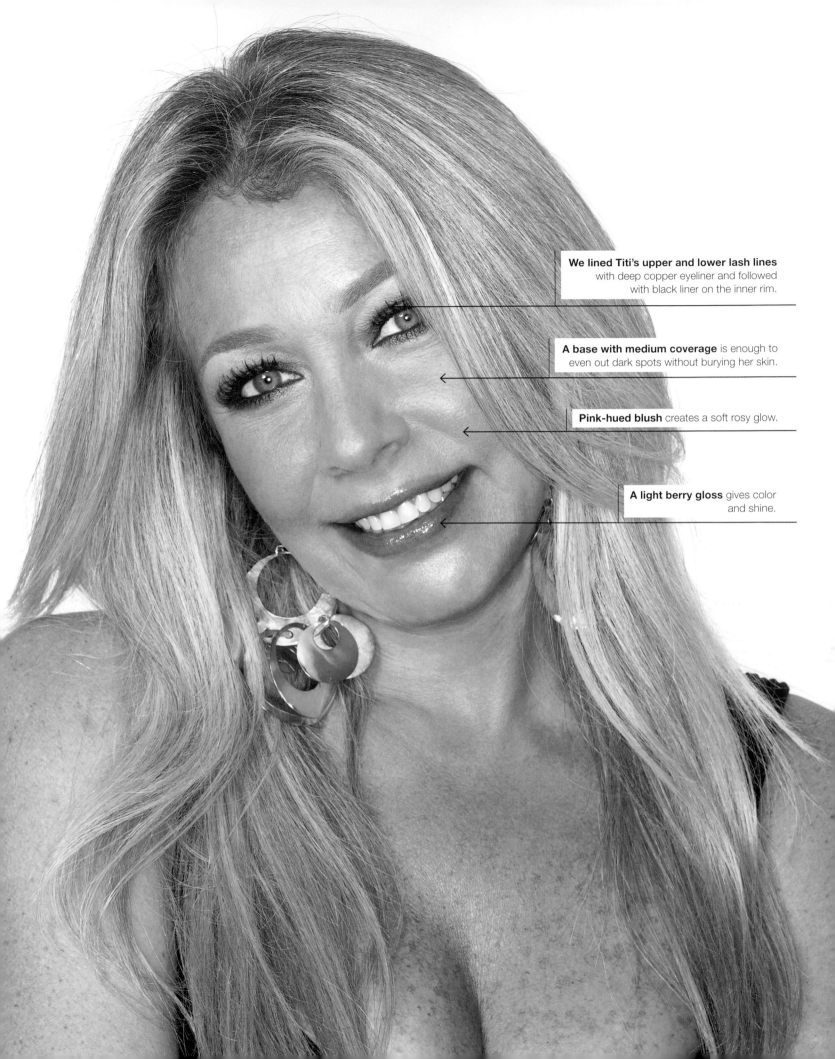

We lined Titi's upper and lower lash lines with deep copper eyeliner and followed with black liner on the inner rim.

A base with medium coverage is enough to even out dark spots without burying her skin.

Pink-hued blush creates a soft rosy glow.

A light berry gloss gives color and shine.

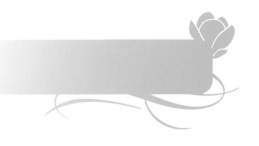

fifties

patricia

Patricia is a Hindu goddess in the body of an Italian girl. New York City, where everyone seems to dress in black, can look like a dark cave—and then there is Patricia in her orange, purple, and green saris and her beautiful nose ring (which I insisted be left in, to be part of her "after" look). Patricia, a yoga instructor, taught me how to breathe, how to receive oxygen into every cell of my being, using the technique and belief system that she not only teaches but lives. It's called viniyoga. Patricia brings me peace and calmness. Besides helping her huge clientele, Patricia teaches yoga to preschoolers on Coney Island. She gives of herself to everybody and has changed my life in so many ways. It was time for her to get something for herself.

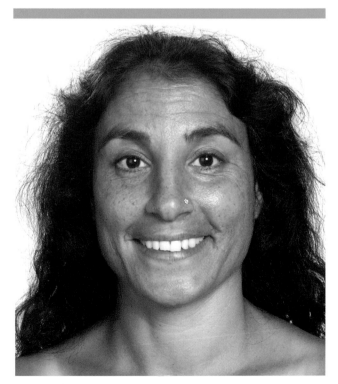

BEFORE Patricia's love of life and the outdoors is obvious, and we wanted to make sure that her makeover enhanced her inner glow.

FACE We applied it with a damp sponge over moisturized skin and paid special attention to her eye area, to be sure we camouflaged any dark circles. To avoid having any makeup settling into or caking the fine lines around Patricia's eyes, we applied eye cream right before we applied an illuminating concealer. The eye cream also ensures that the skin around the eyes remains supple.

CHEEKS We applied bronzer, not blush, with a big, fluffy brush to her cheeks, chin, temples, and forehead and ended with a light brushing on the nose to mimic where the sun hits naturally.

EYES To emphasize and visually enlarge her eyes, we applied a dark eyeliner along the top lid and extended the line outward slightly beyond her lash line. We curled her natural lashes with an eyelash curler and then applied a few individual clusters of fake lashes along the outside edges of her lash line, to heighten the flirty effect. We finished with a light coat of black mascara to "blend" the fake and the real lashes.

LIPS We used a skin-tone lip-liner to give Patricia's lips more definition. A dusty rose gloss on top gave her shine and a hint of color.

HAIR Patricia's lush, long black hair is her signature. We smoothed her hair out using a flat iron. Sweeping it to the side will keep her look fresh and hip.

AFTER Bronzed and beautiful, Patricia is a perfect example of how bronzer is for everyone, not just twenty-year-olds.

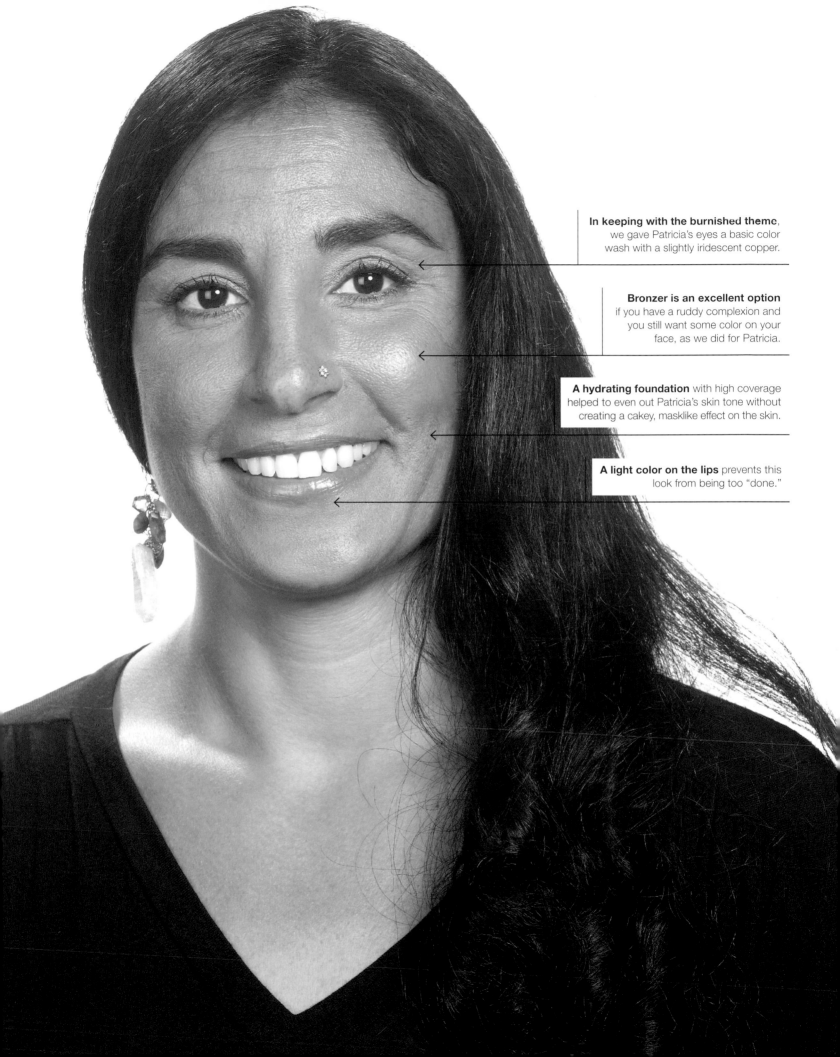

In keeping with the burnished theme, we gave Patricia's eyes a basic color wash with a slightly iridescent copper.

Bronzer is an excellent option if you have a ruddy complexion and you still want some color on your face, as we did for Patricia.

A hydrating foundation with high coverage helped to even out Patricia's skin tone without creating a cakey, masklike effect on the skin.

A light color on the lips prevents this look from being too "done."

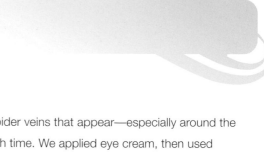

sixty and beyond…

yolanda

The person who came to mind when I wanted to represent the beauty of women sixty and older was my mother. I call her the Mexican Energizer Bunny. She radiates health and happiness. She was very happy to be a part of this book, and I am honored to have her. She is the wind beneath my wings, and I would not be where I am today, writing this book, if it weren't for her courage and energy. She taught me to have confidence, to believe in my dreams, and to never be afraid to express myself no matter how difficult the situation. She is the person who pushes me all the way up, a los cuernos de la luna.

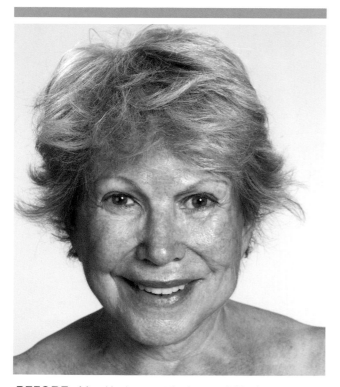

BEFORE Mami looks great for her age! She has a young spirit and a curious, lively mind that keeps her fresh. Her look should reflect this.

FACE We applied a rich cream foundation to smooth out the surface of Mami's skin and to tone down redness and the tiny spider veins that appear—especially around the nose—with time. We applied eye cream, then used brightening concealer under her eyes. We finished with sparing use of loose translucent powder to set her makeup, keeping it light because a too-dry face can lend makeup a heavy, cakey finish.

CHEEKS We applied a soft, warm-toned blush to the apples of Mami's cheeks to bring out her smile. We put shaping powder along her jawline, in the hollows of her cheeks, and on her temples for a slimming effect.

EYES We used pencil to define the basic shape of the brow, and powder to build and fill in the rest then applied a light-colored gel to set the brows. We applied a neutral base color to prepare each eye, then a light-toned highlighter on each brow bone. We opted for a rich walnut brown in the crease and along the top and bottom lash line to frame her eye. Fake lashes helped beef up a sparse lash line. We finished with mascara iy lista!

LIPS We used a cranberry-colored cream lipstick to define Mami's lips and a coordinating lip-liner to hold the color, helping to minimize any potential bleeding of color into the fine lines along the edges of her lips.

HAIR As you can tell, I got my round face from Mami. If you have a cara redonda too, styling your short haircut with more volume at the crown visually elongates the face and slims the cheeks. We dampened Mami's hair, then used a blow-dryer with a small-barrel round brush. You also can use a thickening spray at the roots to add volume, and pomade smoothed lightly over the surface will keep your hair from getting too puffy. Side-swept bangs are also very flattering on most women.

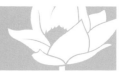

AFTER Ready to go out, turn heads, and kick butt!

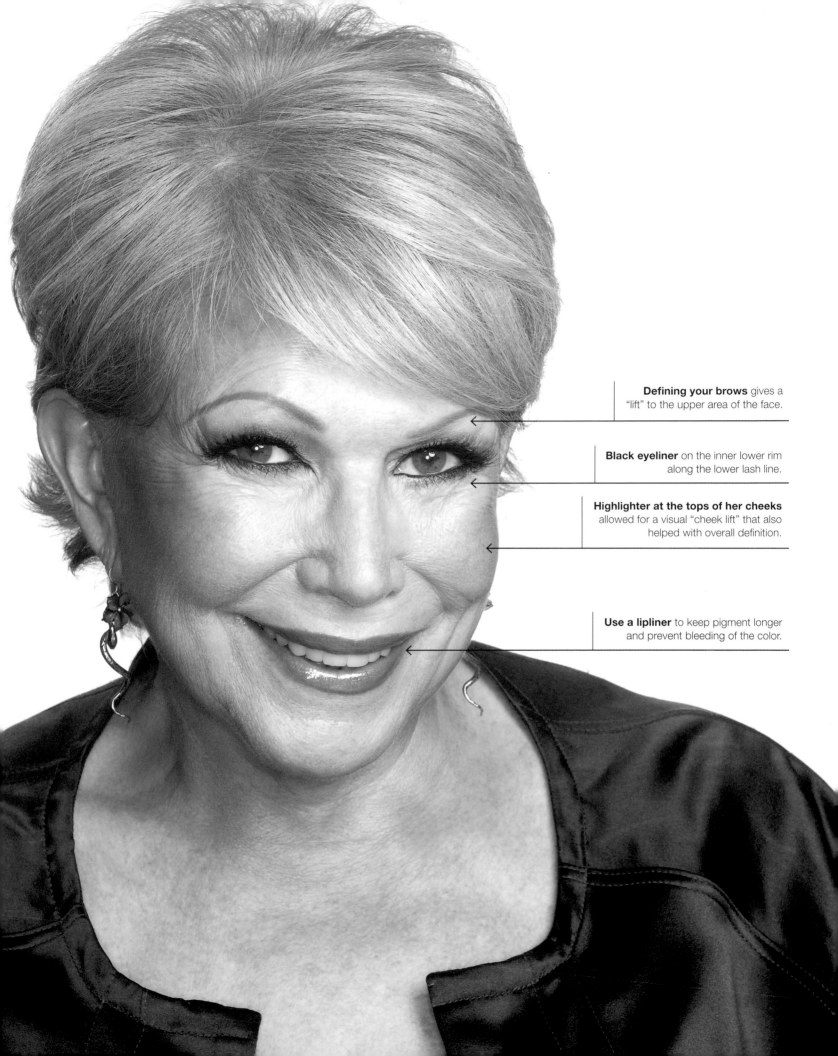

Defining your brows gives a "lift" to the upper area of the face.

Black eyeliner on the inner lower rim along the lower lash line.

Highlighter at the tops of her cheeks allowed for a visual "cheek lift" that also helped with overall definition.

Use a lipliner to keep pigment longer and prevent bleeding of the color.

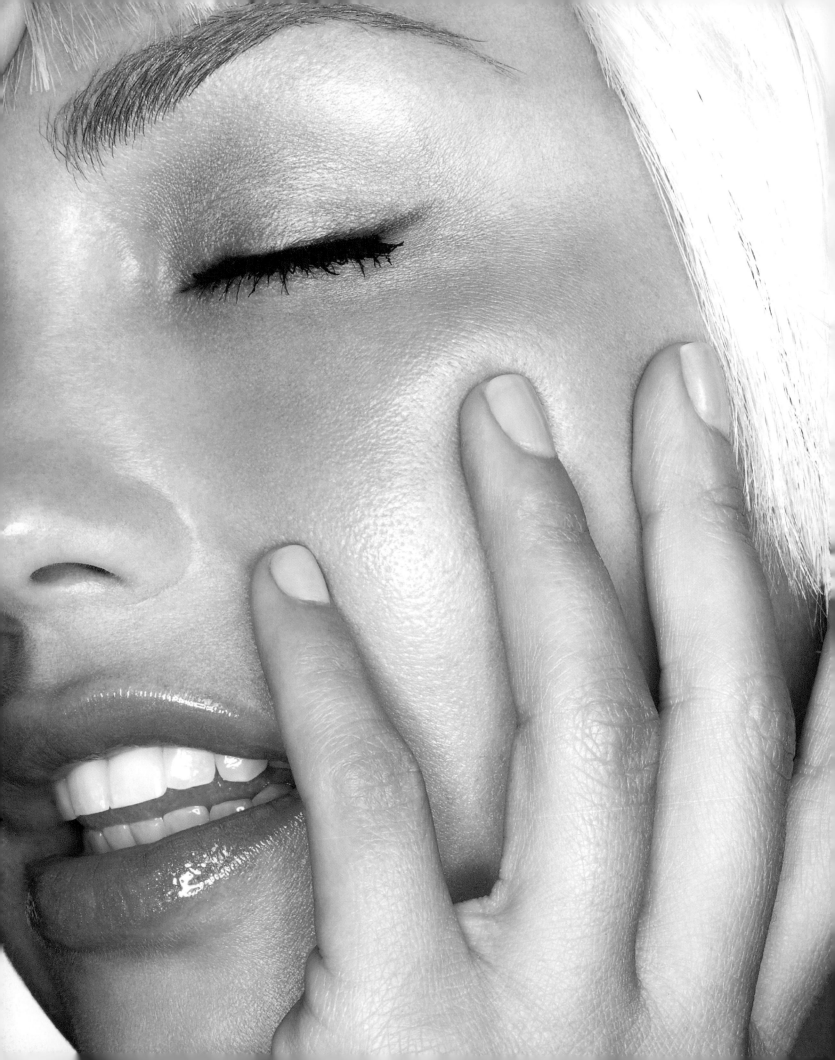

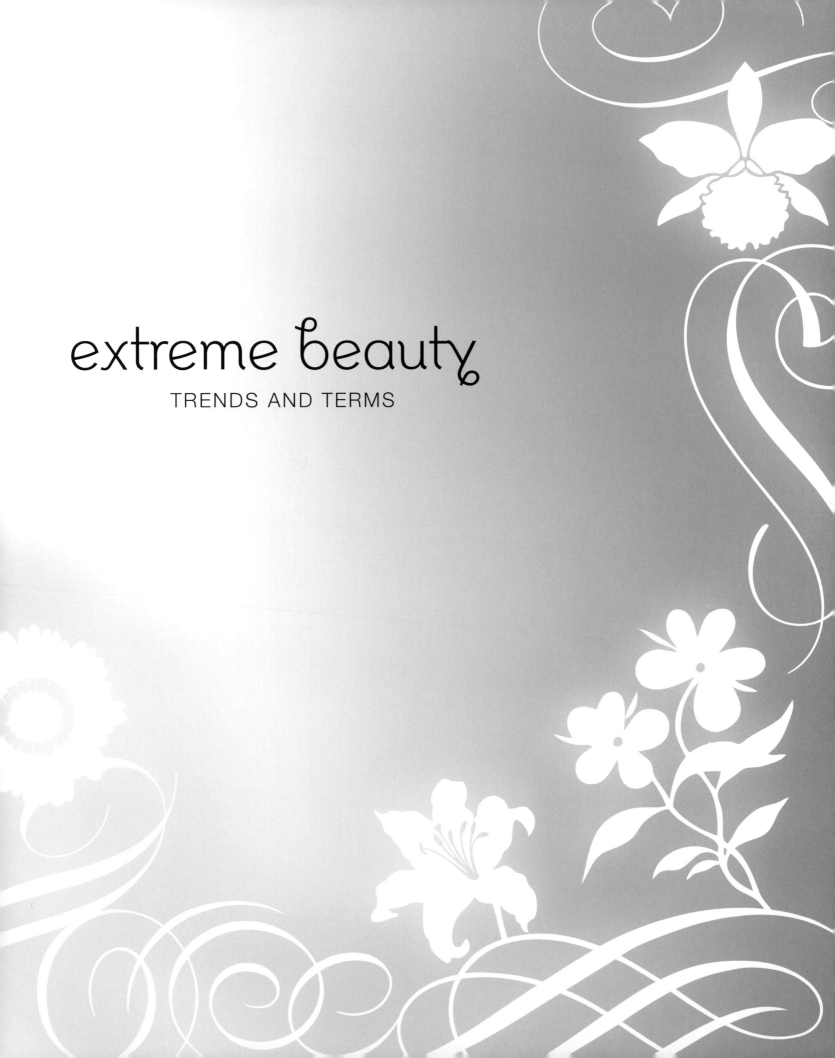

extreme beauty
TRENDS AND TERMS

Listen up, ladies: As a woman who has been to the cutting edge of beauty techniques without actually having to go under the knife, I'm here to tell you: it's not necessary to resort to plastic surgery. Loads of new techniques are out there that offer impressive results. From lash extensions to lasers, I've done it all. One of my favorite moments as a celebrity is when I meet a fan for the first time who tells me I look exactly the way I did when I was on *María la del Barrio*, one of my earliest telenovelas. That's when I know that all of the McDonald's Happy Meals I don't eat (but absolutely adore!) and all of the mojitos I don't drink (well, I'm human, so yes, once in a while I indulge) and all the latest beauty boosters I've tried have paid off.

In this chapter, I'll go over those edgy beauty techniques that you've always been curious about but were afraid to ask. Before we go any further, though, let me tell you that if you want to try any of these things, it is crucial to first investigate the procedure you want to have done and research the doctor you are choosing to administer this procedure. Finding a good doctor is harder than finding information. Try to talk to women who have had the procedure done before, and ask them about their experience. Visit the doctor for a consultation. The consultation should be free: no reputable doctor would charge you for exercising due diligence. If you wouldn't go to a stylist without a positive recommendation from one of your trusted girlfriends, don't even think about letting a stranger put chemicals near your face without the same assurances.

And remember, I recommend you approach any beauty treatment with a sense of curiosity and adventure, but also with a healthy respect for your own instincts and comfort level. It's fun to read about the latest trends for beauty procedures, but there are tons of products out there that can help you look and feel great for less.

body thermage

In this procedure, a doctor uses radio frequency waves to stimulate collagen production and cause the underlying tissues to become taut. During the procedure, which takes a few hours, a topical numbing agent is applied to the area being treated, and you feel a heating sensation followed quickly by a cooling sensation. This process was originally used on the face to help tighten the neck and jowls area. Doctors have recently started to apply thermage to other body parts, and the procedure has become known as the noninvasive tummy tuck, helping tighten panzas that have stretch marks and loose skin. Thermage tightens and contours the tummy because it spurs collagen production in the deep layers of the skin. The results won't be as dramatic as a real tummy tuck, and the procedure can't eliminate stretch marks altogether, but the results from thermage last three to five years. The cost ranges from $1,200 to $2,500, depending on the area you are having treated.

body titan

An alternative to thermage, Body Titan also tightens the skin substantially and increases collagen production. Body Titan uses infrared rays to stimulate collagen production, resulting in a tightening of the skin. It is considered less painful than thermage, but it requires three to five treatments. The cost is $700 to $2,000 per treatment.

botox

This is now the most popular cosmetic procedure in the United States, but its only FDA-approved use is for the forehead. The doctor injects a muscle relaxer into the muscles of the forehead. They cannot contract as they would when you naturally feel shock or surprise. Since the muscles underlying the skin are not moving, the top layer of skin smooths out, causing the eyebrows to appear lifted and you to appear much more, shall we say, serene. Some dermatologists swear that getting regular Botox injections every four to six months can help prevent deeper lines from forming, which is why women in their mid-thirties are turning to it in droves at special "Botox parties." However, Botox has been tested in studies that

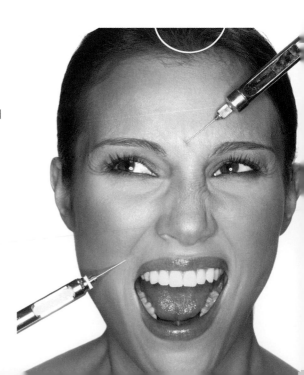

lasted only a period of nine years—not very long at all. Plus, if your doctor injects the Botox into the wrong place, or if the toxin leaks into other areas, you may be left with droopy eyes. Botox wears off after four to six months, which suggests that there won't be any permanent disfiguration. If you are finding that you have to return more often than every four to six months, you should try a different dermatologist. The one you've been going to might be using a diluted form of Botox. If the price you are paying for your botox injections is lower than the going rate (approximately $300 or more per area) then you also have reason to be suspicious.

■ CELEB SECRET REVEALED!

Before there was Botox, there was Scotch tape: Beatrice Sheridan, a director I worked with when I was doing telenovelas, used to have me put a piece of masking tape on my forehead right between my eyebrows. Every time I would furrow my brows, I would feel the Scotch tape there. This literally "trained" me to not furrow my brows and cause wrinkles in my forehead. This is much cheaper, and much less scary, than the needle.

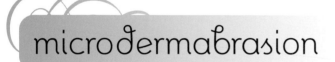

microdermabrasion

This is a high-tech scraping off of the top layer of skin to get to the newer, fresher skin underneath. Tiny aluminum oxide crystals are sprayed against the skin to remove dead skin cells. I had microdermabrasion done to help treat my leftover acne scars. Latinas have to be really careful when considering this procedure: it can leave hyperpigmentation—that is, dark spots—on darker skin tones. For me as a former acne sufferer, it was great. A series of four to six sessions is usually the course of treatment. The cost per session is $150 or more.

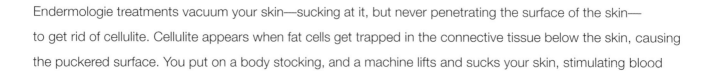

endermologie

Endermologie treatments vacuum your skin—sucking at it, but never penetrating the surface of the skin— to get rid of cellulite. Cellulite appears when fat cells get trapped in the connective tissue below the skin, causing the puckered surface. You put on a body stocking, and a machine lifts and sucks your skin, stimulating blood

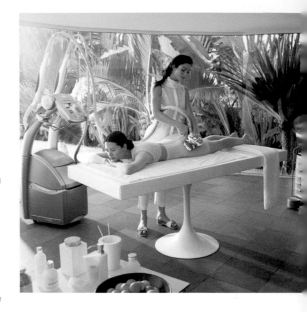

flow to help minimize the appearance of cellulite. With Endermologie, the cellulite is gone for as long as you do the treatment regularly. If you stop, the cottage-cheese-like surface returns, although not as noticeably. Endermologie can also take some inches off the body, but it's not as though you can eat unlimited rice and beans. No one has invented a machine to allow that. You still have to take care of yourself.

I go through phases of doing Endermologie regularly, then taking it easy for a while. I actually bought my own machine so I could do it at home, because I, like most women, hate that icky dimpled skin that just never goes away, no matter how much dieting and exercise you do. Endermologie costs $80 to $100 per session. You will need at least fourteen sessions twice a week to see results that could last for several months, but are not permanent.

fotofacial

This treatment uses pulses of hot laser light to help combat flushed redness, minimize the appearance of big pores, remove broken capillaries, and tighten the skin overall. The technician or dermatologist applies a thick gel to your face and, using light settings that are appropriate to your skin tone and skin concerns, pulses a laser onto the surface of your skin. It takes three or four treatments to notice changes in skin tone, but it evens out your skin tone very nicely. The fotofacial also stimulates collagen production, which should cause a slight tightening of the skin. The effects should last as long as you religiously keep your treated skin covered with sunscreen. You need to space the treatments over three to four months. The cost is about $200 per treatment.

gentle waves

Gentle Waves uses low-energy light panels, under which you sit for a treatment that lasts forty-five minutes. Pulses of the light are thought to help slow the aging process of the skin by stimulating collagen production. The procedure also decreases inflammation of the skin and helps to even out skin tone. Gentle Waves treatments are often combined with two other treatments, such as a gentle microdermabrasion or a peel. When done in conjunction with other methods it is called a triad treatment. One Gentle Waves treatment alone can cost $100 or more, and treatments are usually performed twice a month.

injectable fillers

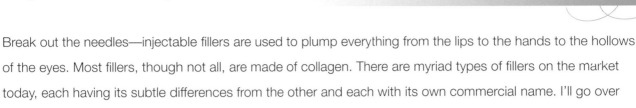

Break out the needles—injectable fillers are used to plump everything from the lips to the hands to the hollows of the eyes. Most fillers, though not all, are made of collagen. There are myriad types of fillers on the market today, each having its subtle differences from the other and each with its own commercial name. I'll go over some of the most popular ones.

Restalyne and CosmoDerm temporarily plump up the facial lines that form around the mouth (called nasio-labial folds). They also can be used to fill the hollows of the eyes, and—most famously—to plump the lips. Their results last a few months. Sculptra and Radiesse are two newer types of fillers whose results, the manufacturers claim, last for years. Sculptra also is said to help spur your own collagen production.

Some fillers use hyaluronic acid, a substance that naturally occurs in the skin. It has wonderful hydrating properties and is used as an ingredient in many expensive skin creams. It is also the main ingredient in a group of injectables with the names Restalyne, Hylaform, Juvederm, and Captique. It hydrates and plumps with no known adverse effects, and it also helps diminish dark circles under the eyes. Restalyne lasts about six months and is used for moderate to deep wrinkles. It costs $550 per injection. Hylaform does not last as long as Restalyne, but it costs the same. The benefit? There is less post-injection swelling with Hylaform, which makes it better for the queasy.

Many dermatologists offer injections at their offices, and an increasing number of spas are offering the procedure as well. At a spa, the actual injection may be administered by an aesthetician as opposed to a doctor. Make sure you understand how much experience the person has before you agree to go under the needle. And remember: no fillers are permanent, and they all induce varying levels of discomfort. You are, after all, having something injected into your face.

lasers

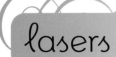

Lasers are some of the newest dermatological weapons on the block, and there are new variations of laser treatments coming out seemingly each day. Resurfacing lasers, or ablative lasers—not the nonablative laser used in fotofacials—target brown spots, discoloration, enlarged pores, and broken capillaries. Lasers use infrared light to stimulate collagen production in the deeper layers of the skin. Fraxel is one popular new option. This laser process creates tiny wounds in the upper layers of the skin. As the skin repairs itself and

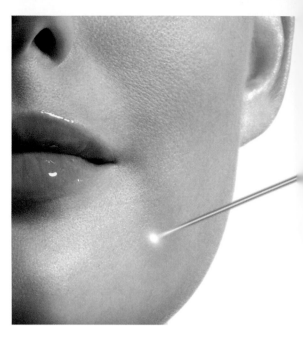

collagen is produced, brown spots and discoloration disappear while texture, firmness, and tightness improve. The treatment causes no redness or oozing, as the older laser treatments or chemical peels do, but it will make you look like you've ignored my sun-protection advice, because you will appear to have a really bad sunburn. Just tell your coworkers you flew to Miami for the weekend. Wait a few weeks, and they will marvel at the glow your weekend getaway gave you! You will need up to six treatments over eight to twelve weeks, depending on how much corrective work is needed. The cost is $500 to $1,500 per treatment.

lash extensions

Individual synthetic lashes are literally bonded to your current lashes in this procedure, glued strand by strand using a high-powered bonding agent that lasts up to two months. It takes time (around two hours) and can be pricey, anywhere from $300 to $500 at a reputable spa or salon. The process is not painful, but it isn't particularly comfortable, either, since you have to sit still with your eyes closed for so long and have someone touching and working around your delicate lash line. The individual strands do eventually

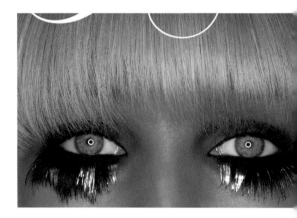

start falling out, and some places that offer lash extensions will do touch-ups to keep your set looking as fresh as possible. Eyelash extensions should last up to four weeks. In terms of upkeep, you can't get your lashes wet for two days after the procedure, and you have to keep oily eye makeup remover away from your lashes at all costs. But once you have the extensions, you can put aside your eyelash curler and your mascara, because you'll have come-hither flirty lashes that won't need either.

peels

Trichloroacetic (TCA, for short), glycolic, salicylic, and lactic acid are all different types of acid peels for the skin. During a peel, a chemical solution lifts away the outermost layer of skin, destroying damaged cells. It's like an alpha hydroxy cream on steroids. As the old cells slough off and the new skin emerges, you will shed like a snake for about a week. The peels will fade brown spots and tighten skin texture. If you want a chemical peel, get one only under the supervision of a doctor who knows what he or she is doing: if the solution is left on too long, it could leave you scarred. A series of three to six peels is usually recommended. Glycolic or salicylic acid peels cost $100 to $200 per peel. TCA peels cost around $250, depending on the amount of TCA in the formula.

podologia

I first tried this procedure in Venezuela, and I have yet to see it offered here in the States. Podologia is a pedicure treatment in which a machine that looks like a floor refinisher you get at Home Depot is used on calluses and any other hardened areas of the feet, top or bottom. I kid you not when I tell you that it restores your feet to the softness of a newborn's, leaving them exquisitely touchable and beautiful! I think that if enough Latin women request it, some spa somewhere in the United States will get the machine and start offering the procedure here. Pídelo!

threading

Threading removes unwanted hair by catching it up in a tightly wound, double-coiled cotton string that an aesthetician quickly rolls over your skin. It's renowned for its precision: hair is removed in a straight, razor-sharp line. Threading removes hair from the roots just like waxing does, but without the discomfort of having hot wax applied to your face. The pain level is about the same as that of waxing or tweezing. Some women use the process all over their face, but its most popular use is on the brows: it will give you eyebrows worthy of a Bollywood film star. Since hair is being removed from the roots, you will need to rethread about as often as you need to retweeze or rewax your brows. Threading is very affordable, from $5 to $15 per treatment. This is a low-risk walk on beauty's wild side.

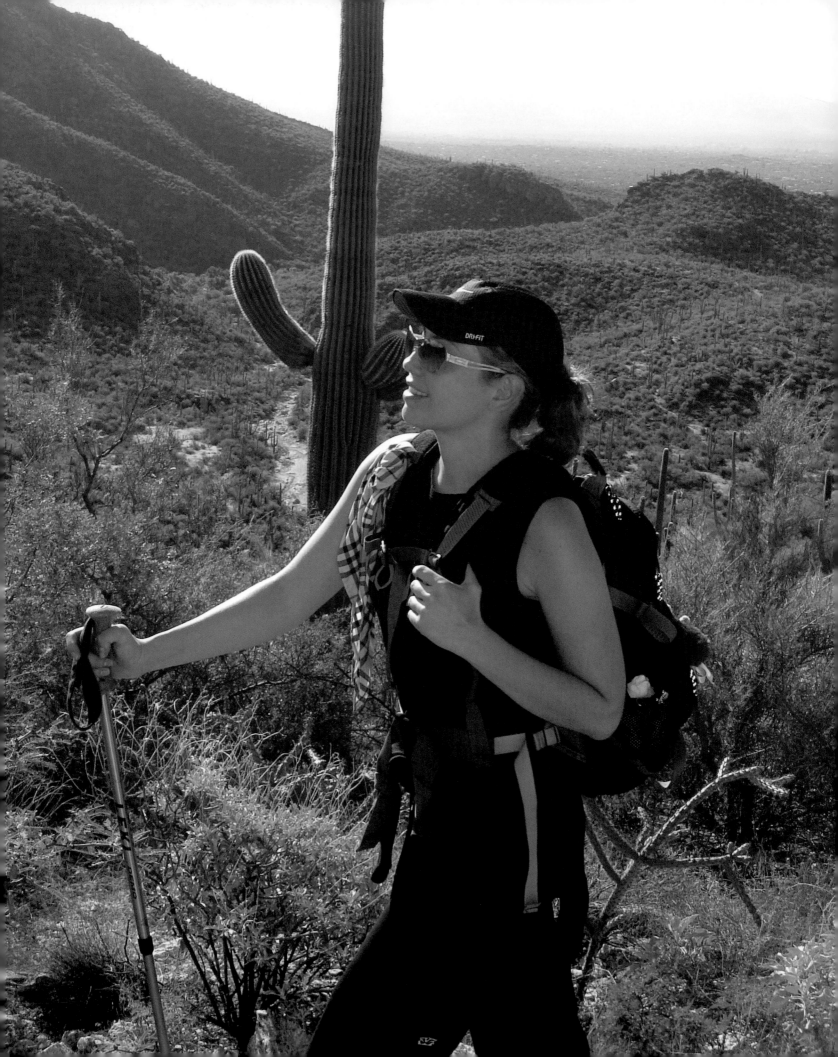

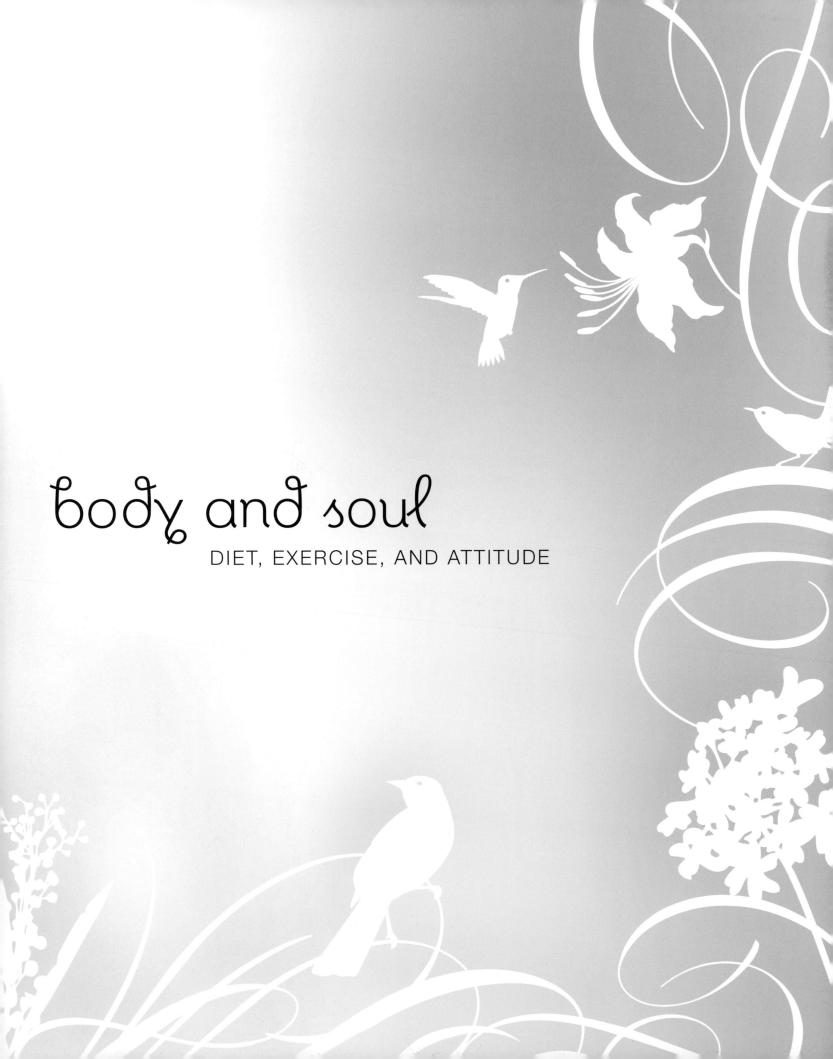

body and soul

DIET, EXERCISE, AND ATTITUDE

¡Atrévete! There is no word in English that accurately captures the sense of urgency, boldness, and fearlessness that this command conveys. Yet this word embodies the spirit of this book as a whole. We are—each and every one of us—beautiful, sexy, and authentic. It is simply a matter of finding the ways to express these aspects of ourselves and freeing ourselves from the mental barriers that may inhibit our best qualities. If you can imagine your life as a house, then you can see this time in your life as an opportunity to renovate it, so it reflects to the world the person you are within.

I have a very active spiritual life, one that influences me on many levels. I believe that we all have a very personal relationship with God. Whether you are Jewish, Christian, Muslim, or pray every day to la madre tierra or to the sun, you have to do what clicks with and comforts your soul and your spirit. In this chapter, I will share this very personal part of myself, touching on the various beliefs that inspire and guide me in my everyday life. This section of the book is the heart of the entire project. It encompasses the importance of a positive mental attitude when it comes to facing daily stressors, simple breathing exercises, my practice of yoga, and how what you put into your body affects what you see on the outside.

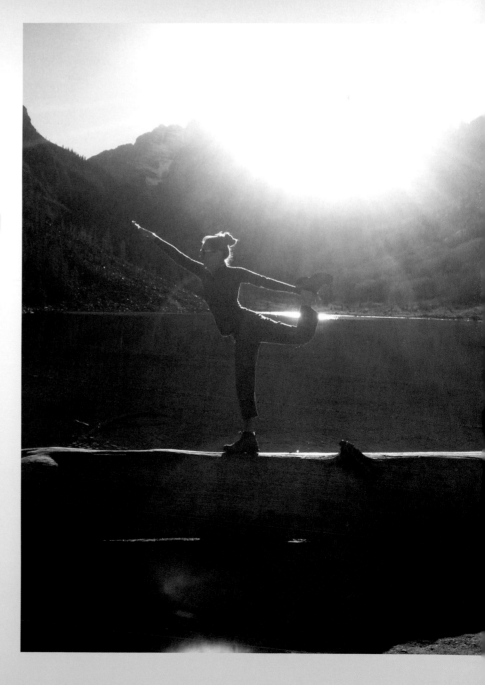

auras, attitude, and assessment

If there is one thing that is true about so many Latinas, it is that we share a positive mental attitude . . . and a flair for the dramatic. Melodramatic tendencies and a love of telenovelas aside, if we did not possess our positive mental attitudes, we, and the women who came before us, would not have taken the leap of faith it takes to change our lives forever. We would not have believed that our lives were *ours* to shape and direct.

I try to surround myself only with people who are positive. I believe that people have energy fields, and that these energy fields can be positive or negative, depending on how the person sees and interacts with the world around her. This energy field is the person's aura, and each and every one of us has our own unique aura. Auras are invisible, but you can get a sense of a person's aura by observing things about him: his mood, his stance, just the general vibe he gives off. You can feel it when you are around a person with a positive aura and an optimistic mental attitude. Being with her is energizing, inspiring, and fun. Just the same, you can feel it when you are around someone with a negative aura: spend time with him and you will feel drained and listless, even if you haven't done anything particularly strenuous or difficult.

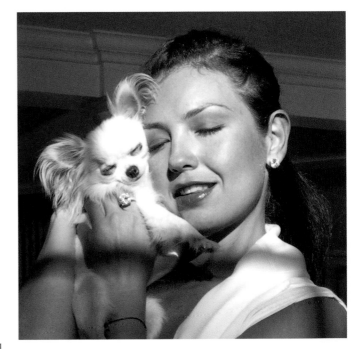

Now don't get me wrong: I have my bad days. We all do. Not everyone's energy field is going to be radiant and luminous all the time. So I don't immediately judge or dismiss people who might just be having a bad day, and I don't think other people should either. I do, however, take into account what my instincts tell me about a person. As a public person, I am always aware that no matter what I do, there will be critics and complainers who have something to say about me. In stressful situations, I use my breathing techniques and prayer to keep me centered and focused. Also, when I am stressed out, I love to do different things. I enjoy going to toy stores and watching kids as they experience pure pleasure and curiosity at the things that surround them. I'll go to a pet store and watch the little animals and the reactions they elicit from humans. Or, like I mentioned before, I like to hit the beauty aisle at the drugstore or stop in to browse at Sephora. I am always curious about the latest and greatest beauty innovations, and looking at all the aisles packed with cool stuff gets me out of my own head and thinking about what I want to try, what other women are drawn to, and how making oneself feel pretty is such a powerful way to feel better.

The other thing I have done repeatedly throughout my career is give back to the community. As much as you will see me at awards shows and movie premieres and concerts, you also will see me at charity events and taking part in public service activities. My favorite charities are the Robin Hood Foundation and March of Dimes. I regularly do events with all of the charities I can and include them when I am launching new projects. Helping other people makes me learn new things and appreciate a new world. It gives my own life greater meaning. When I am giving, I am no longer worrying about my problems. Going out and volunteering your time lets other people know that there is help and that we are not alone. I am passionate about the March of Dimes because it helps children, the people in our society who have no voice. Helping others gives you a purpose in this life. It makes you feel productive and good about your life and yourself.

One exercise I do that helps me understand myself better only requires a pen, a piece of paper, and the willingness to look at oneself with love and curiosity and without judging yourself too harshly. Separate a piece of paper into three columns. At the top of one, write "I like"; on top of the second, write "I will change"; and at the top of the third column, write, "I will rescue." In the first column I would write what I like about myself: "My happiness, my creativity, my honesty." In column two, I would write what I will change about myself: "My impatience, my explosive character, my behavioral patterns that no longer help me." In the last column I would write about the side of myself that I want to revive: "The adventurous little girl, my curiosity for new ideas, and my sense of surprise."

I look at all of the columns to understand myself better, but I seriously try to work on the elements of the second column. With each aspect of myself that I want to change, I look deeper into myself and I analyze what triggers these caracteristicas. Then I proactively try to change these things.

I believe that being happy or unhappy is an active decision we make repeatedly every day. So I make that choice. I choose to be happy. *I choose* to make myself a better person. And I choose to also recognize what is good about me as well.

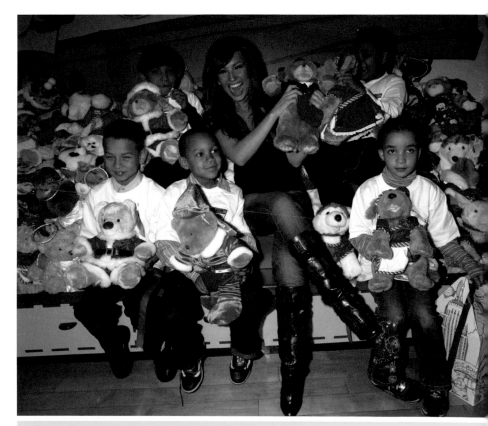

I have so much fun any time I am with the kids of the Police Athletic League. Here I am at a Build a Bear Event right before the Holidays.

breathing basics

I was a grown woman before I finally learned how to breathe properly. I was taught by my wonderful yoga teacher, Patricia. Taking a breath of air is instinctive, something we do without thinking and something we must do in order to survive. But do you want to survive, or do you want to thrive? In order to thrive, you need to learn how to breathe the right way, by taking conscious breaths and understanding how breathing brings oxygen to every cell of your body. Oxygen is life itself, it is energy, and it is everywhere. You must start by breathing slowly and deeply, using your lungs and expanding your stomach, not your chest.

The following breathing exercise will help calm you, giving you a moment of serenity in the midst of the all of the must-dos of daily life. Try it when you're feeling stressed, when you can't fall asleep, when you're riding the elevator down from a long day at work—whenever you need to refocus your energy and feel calm.

Inhale through your nose as deeply as you can for a count of five. In your mind picture your lungs filling with air to their maximum capacity. To truly breathe deeply, you must allow your belly to expand.

Hold the breath for another count of five.

Exhale through your mouth, expelling all of the air in your lungs. You will exhale for much longer than you inhaled, up to a count of ten.

Concentrate on this slow and steady exhalation, imagining all of the old air leaving your body and being sent out into the universe.

Turn the exercise into a meditative experience by imagining as you breathe in that serenity and clarity are entering your body and filling it as the air is filling your lungs. As you exhale, imagine that all your stress and worries are being released with that old air, making a space for new things in your life to come.

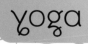 yoga

I am sure many of you have already heard about yoga, even if you have not tried it. Sure, it may seem strange: why would someone want to fold herself into the shape of a pretzel and stay there for a minute or more? But I have been doing yoga for more than ten years now, and I consider it one of the greatest gifts I have been given. The practice of Sivananda yoga—one of the oldest forms—and viniyoga has given me a boost in energy while at the same time helping me to relax. I try to do some yoga poses daily, and whenever I get the chance, I take a class. This can be hard to do, what with my travel schedule, but I try to do it as often as I can.

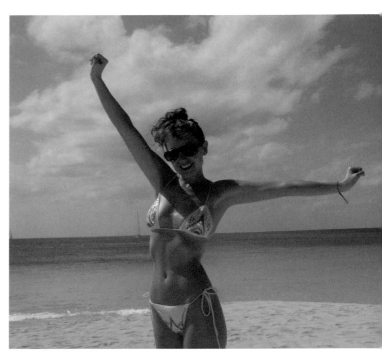

There are many different types of yoga practices, some with histories that go back hundreds or thousands of years. The style of yoga I practice is called viniyoga, and what distinguishes it from other types of yoga is that it puts a tremendous amount of emphasis on breathing and on the self. Viniyoga is excellent for all levels of yoga practice, but it is especially great for beginners, because the poses are adapted to each individual's ability. A good yoga instructor will take you through poses and simultaneous breathing exercises that will help you release stress. If you need to reconnect and refocus, the poses and breathing exercises will help you to center yourself, to find inner quiet focus. Yoga puts as much emphasis on the mental as it does on the physical. It is a true coming together of the body, mind, and spirit.

You don't necessarily need to practice yoga to feel the flow. Find an exercise that centers you, something that makes you feel relaxed and whole. Whatever works for you personally. Maybe running puts you in the zone. Or long walks listening to your favorite music. You don't have to join a gym and commit to a ferocious workout schedule to get the benefits of physical activity. Walking, stretching, dancing—and great sex!—are all excellent ways to get your body moving.

I also like to try different things like pilates or a new machine at the gym. It keeps my body toned and my work-out interesting.

letting go

I started doing this practice when I was seven years old: I write letters to God, telling him everything that is on my mind, including my worries, my questions, my embarrassing thoughts, and my fears. Then I put the letter in a balloon, fill the balloon with helium, and release the balloon out into the atmosphere. This exercise is about letting go. You are giving over control to your higher power and relieving yourself of the responsibility to change everything, or to carry the weight of the world on your shoulders. A friend once told me to "let go and let God."

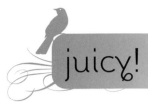

juicy!

This is a beauty book, not a diet book (I'll write that one later). But just as I would not be comfortable writing a beauty book without saying that a great set of eyebrows is as important as a great mind-set, I would feel like I was ignoring my own beliefs—and an ever-growing pile of research—if I didn't talk a little bit about how what you put into your body makes a big difference in what you see in the mirror.

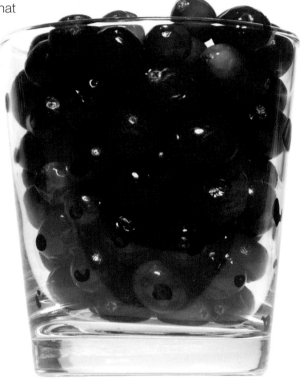

I don't believe in crazy diets or random food fads, although I do like to try new things. I'm like most women in that Monday through Friday, I try to keep a routine of eating a healthful, balanced diet. During the weekends, I give myself more leeway—and flan! But I try not to go overboard, because there is nothing worse than post-pig-out depression. It's just not worth it.

One little trick I have for getting back on track—or staying there— is juicing. No, I don't go on juice fasts; I make juice concoctions. They are great especially when I am feeling too rushed to eat a salad, or when I want to cleanse my system. Here are my two favorite recipes:

popeye juice

This is a veggie drink, but you can mix in some fruit juice to make it more palatable.

TAKE EVERY GREEN THING you can find in your refrigerator—spinach, celery, pears, green apples, even jalapeños. Add some color if you dare: beets, ginger, a garlic clove.

LIQUEFY them all in a food processor.

DRINK. Pinch your nose, don't think too much about it, and toss that juice back like you're downing a shot of tequila. Popeye juice doesn't give you a hangover—I promise!

detoxifying juice

Ideally, you will use juices you have squeezed or blended yourself rather than concentrate, which is high in sugar and preservatives, but regular juice from the carton will do.

ONE CUP orange juice.

ONE CUP pineapple juice.

ONE TEASPOON fresh, finely grated ginger.

BLEND in a blender with ice for a frothy smoothie effect.

DRINK!

tips for a healthful diet

I try to eat in moderation, incorporating proven beauty-boosters such as the following into my diet:

❋ Oily fish such as wild salmon, which contains essential fatty acids that give skin a glow.

❋ Water, which keeps the skin hydrated from within and flushes out toxins that cause, among other things, acne.

❋ Green veggies, which are high in the antioxidants that fight aging free radicals.

❋ Whole grains, such as whole wheat bread, brown rice, quinoa, and avena.

❋ Fruits. All kinds, all colors, every day.

The foods I avoid include:

❋ Processed foods with tons of chemicals I find hard to pronounce.

❋ Too much caffeine. As a diuretic, caffeine dehydrates the body, which in turn will dry my skin.

❋ White, refined flours, which not only leave me feeling hungry shortly after eating them, but also make me puffy and bloated. These flours can contribute to skin inflammation as well.

❋ Saturated fats.

❋ White, refined sugar.

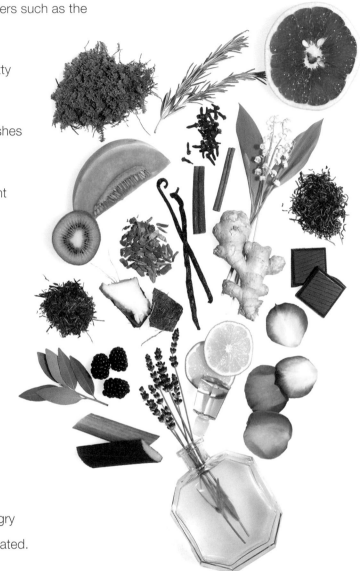

Because I lead such a busy life, crossing time zones and changing seasons the way some people go on their daily commute, I can't always be sure that I will get all of the vitamins and minerals my body needs to stay strong and healthy. I absolutely swear by supplements as a great way to improve overall health and the appearance of the hair, skin, and nails. Here are some you might want to consider:

VITAMINS C AND E, ALPHA-LIPOIC ACID, GREEN TEA, AND COQ10 These are all antioxidants, which help you fight off the free radicals in the environment that cause aging. They help maintain your collagen and elastin (your skin's own plumpers and hydrators), and they help slow the development of fine lines. Add antioxidants to your diet, too, by eating tons of green veggies and drinking green tea.

B VITAMINS Besides boosting energy, B vitamins help promote strong hair and nails. A deficiency of B vitamins in your diet will result in brittle nail tips and slack, unresponsive skin.

OMEGA-3 FATTY ACIDS I take three omega supplements a day every day. Omegas are linked to so many benefits, from lowering cholesterol to staving off depression. This supplement is a must-have and completely familiar to anyone who remembers taking spoonfuls of aceite de bacalao when she was growing up. Trust me: supplements taste much better. The latest buzz suggests that omegas help to calm skin irritation and even might help assuage acne, psoriasis, and eczema.

PROBIOTICS Getting your probiotics is so easy, it almost feels like you are cheating: just eat a serving of organic yogurt every day. Probiotics help to balance the yeast in your body. Yeast overgrowth can result in lackluster skin and even shedding, scaling skin. You can take probiotics in supplement form if yogurt is hard on your stomach.

ZINC I keep zinc lozenges on hand and take them at the first sign of a cold. Zinc also benefits the skin: it can regulate the skin's oil production and reduce acne flare-ups.

thalia tips

❋ Find time for yourself

❋ Think positive thoughts

❋ Give back to the community

❋ Follow a healthful food plan that works for you

❋ Drink lots of water

❋ Use the tips in this book

❋ Take on the world!

So now I have given you the tools to fulfill your own maximum beauty potential. Now you know that lasting beauty is born from within, from positive thoughts and from positive actions. The rest is like the ornaments on a Christmas tree: they sparkle and shine, but they are nothing if they are not on a healthy tree.

Bring beauty to every aspect of your life by embracing change and being bold. Don't be afraid to try the new things that inspire you. Porque vida, solo hay una, cariño.

Mucho amor y mucha luz,

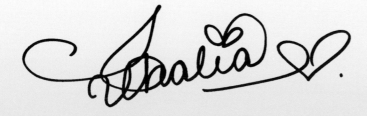

acknowledgments

Grateful acknowledgment to . . .

Our photographers and their teams:

RICHARD MCLAREN
Liselle McReynolds, Michael Labica, Todd Stone, and Frank Roller

ALEX CAO
Jen Joyce Davis, Hiroki Sakamoto, and Bonnie Winston

GEORGE HOLZ
Alexis Tolbert

KEVIN MAZUR
Everyone at Wireimage, especially Justin Weiss,
Rodrigo Varela, Lester Cohen, Gregg Deguire, and Dimitrious Kambouris

ALBERTO TOLOT
Dominique Cole

MICHAEL BIONDO

TORKIL GUDNASON
Judy Casey

MARK LIDDELL

CARLOS SOMONTE

ALFONSO PEREZ BUTRONE

STEVEN SHAW
Icon Photo: Kendra Kabasele and Anna Lambrix

JIMMY IENNER JR.

ANTOINE VERGLAS
Anouck Bertin

STEVE SANDS

Our makeup artists:
Sidney Jamilla
Billy B
Thalia Sodi
Alfonso Waithsman
Clorinda Vitale
Lucky
Shoukefeh Azary

Our hairstylists:
Luis Beltran / Blinkmanagement.com
Peter Butler
Joaquin Hortal
Luis Guillermo
Henry Ospina

Our stylists:
Eric Archibald
David Zambrana
Cory Parker

Our models:
Next Model Management: Kristeen Arnold, Agbani Darego, Natalia Luchinina
Veronica Acosta
Christina Anderson
Yana Radha
Jennifer Vidal
Kristina Collado

Our contributing experts and their affiliations:
Amy E. Newberger, M.D., Founder, Dermatology Consultants of Westchester, author of
Looking Good at Any Age
David Colbert, M.D., Founder, New York Dermatology Group
Joy Bauer, MS, RD, CDN, Joy Bauer Nutrition

Our generous product donors:
M•A•C Cosmetics and Christine Serrão
Mally Beauty and Mally Roncal and Jim Enderato

Our production coordinators:
Mark Mulvey and Christian Martin

A very special thank-you to Daisy Fuentes for her support, graciousness, and infectious energy; Petra Nemcova for her kindness and inspiration; and Gloria Estefan for her loyal friendship and love.

A special thank-you to Lisette Lorenzo at EMI Music for her artful eye and dedication.

And to everyone at Chronicle Books for their enthusiasm and hard work, especially Jodi Warshaw, Kate Prouty, Aya Akazawa, River Jukes-Hudson, Doug Ogan, and Tera Killip.

And, of course, to Tommy Mottola, Belén Aranda-Alvarado, Joanne Oriti, EMI Music, Virgin Records, *Ocean Drive En Español*, *Glamour Latinoamerica*, Peggy Regis L.Ac., P.C., Yudelka Marin, Patricia Sanzone, Yolanda Miranda, Ernestina Sodi, Ruth Roche, Denise Markey, Rita Hazan, Troy Surrat, Matine, Rebecca Restreppo, Oribe, Laurentius Purnama, Roberto DiCuia, Kenmark Eyewear, Hershey's, Gina Eppolito, LPG One, Carol's Daughter, Kim Jackwerth, Mariela Perez, Rachel Turner, Rob Kos, and Nora Jacobs.

Love and thanks to all of you who have come to all of my signings and events. Your support over the years means the world to me. Love you all!

index

photo credits

Cover and pages 5, 28, 32, 46 (lower right), 48, 52, 55 (upper right), 81, 88, 90, 92-93, 136, 144-148, 162, and 165 photographs © by Richard McLaren.

Pages 2 and 10 photographs © by Torkil Gudnason (courtesy EMI Music).

Pages 13, 18, 50, 107 (upper right), 188, 191-192, and 195 photographs courtesy Thalia Sodi.

Pages 14, 16, 17 (upper right), 21, 25-27, 29-31, 33, 38-40, 43-45, 46 (upper right), 47, 53-54, 55 (lower left), 56-57, 59-61, 65-68, 71-72, 86, 87 (top left and lower right), 95, 100-101, 105-106, 107 (lower right), 108-109, 113, 118, 120, 122, 124, 126, 128, 130, 138, 140, 142, 156, 161, 166-178, 182, 186, and 196-197 photographs © by Alex Cao.

Pages 17 (lower left) and 34 photographs © by Michael Biondo.

Pages 20, 62, 96, and 104 photographs © by George Holz.

Pages 22 and 87 (lower left) photographs © by Mark Liddell (courtesy Virgin Records/EMI Music).

Page 51 photograph © by Alfonso Perez Butrone.

Pages 70, 74, and 99 photograph © by Alberto Tolot.

Page 79 photograph © by Torkil Gudnason.

Page 84 photograph © by Carlos Somonte.

Page 85 (upper right) photograph © by Alberto Tolot (courtesy of Ocean Drive En Español).

Page 85 (left) photographs © by Antoine Verglas.

Pages 103 and 184 photographs © courtesy LPG One, Inc.

Pages 110-111 photographs © by George Holz (courtesy EMI Music).

Page 114 photograph © courtesy EMI Music.

Page 132 photograph © by Steve Shaw (Icon Photo International).

Pages 134 and 155 (upper) photographs © by Kevin Mazur (courtesy Wire Image).

Page 152 (upper) photograph © by Jimmy Ienner, Jr.

Page 152 (lower) photographs © courtesy Ocean Drive En Español.

Page 153 photograph © by Rodrigo Varela (courtesy Wire Image).

Page 154 (upper) photograph courtesy Wire Image.

Page 154 (lower) photograph © by Gregg Deguire (courtesy Wire Image).

Page 155 (lower) photograph © by Dimitrius Kambouris (courtesy Wire Image).

Page 193 photograph © by Steve Sands.